Models of
Brain Injury
Rehabilitation

The Johns Hopkins Series in Contemporary Medicine and Public Health

also of interest in this series:
Neuropsychological Rehabilitation after Brain Injury, by George P. Prigatano and Others

Models of
Brain Injury
Rehabilitation

Edited by

RODGER LL. WOOD

and

PETER EAMES

The Johns Hopkins University Press
Baltimore

Published in the United States of America by
The Johns Hopkins University Press
701 West 40th Street
Baltimore, Maryland 21211

Library of Congress Catalog Card Number 88–39621

ISBN 0–8018–3818–5

Printed and bound in Great Britain

Contents

Contributors

Sheldon Berrol, Associate Clinical Professor and Chief of Physical Medicine and Rehabilitation, San Francisco General Hospital, USA.

John Bryden, Community Medicine Specialist, Information Services Unit, Greater Glasgow Health Board, UK.

Peter Eames, Consultant Neuropsychiatrist, Burden Neurological Hospital, Stoke Lane, Stapleton, Bristol, UK.

Chris Evans, Consultant in Rehabilitation Medicine, Royal Cornwall Hospital (City), Infirmary Hill, Truro, Cornwall, UK.

Scott Goll, Director, Case Management Systems, Neurocare, Corporate Headquarters, 1001 Galaxy Way, Suite 400, Concord, CA 94520, USA.

William Haffey, Director of Research, New Medico Inc., 78 Maplewood Shops, Northampton, MA 01060, USA.

Keith Hawley, Behavioural Coordinator, Transitional Living Center, Casa Colina Hospital, North Garey Avenue, Pomona, CA 91767, USA.

Mark Johnston, Senior Research Manager, New Medico Inc., 78 Maplewood Shops, Northampton, MA 01060, USA.

Betty Skidmore, Senior Clinical Psychologist, Blantyre, Truro Road, St Austell, Cornwall, UK.

Reg Talbott, Director, Headway, The National Head Injuries Association, 200 Mansfield Road, Nottingham NG1 3HX, UK.

Barbara Wilson, Senior Lecturer, University Rehabilitation Unit, Southampton General Hospital, Tremona Road, Southampton, UK.

Rodger Ll. Wood, Clinical Director, Brain Injury Rehabilitation Service, Casa Colina Hospital for Rehabilitation Medicine, Pomona, CA 91767, USA.

Preface

The growth of brain injury rehabilitation over the past 8 years has resulted in a greater awareness of a need for specialization in treatment methods, appropriate to the needs of brain-injured patients. Until recently, brain injury rehabilitation lacked a scientific foundation upon which research could develop, individual patients be properly evaluated, and treatment procedures implemented. A fund of knowledge which informs the clinician about the probable recovery process and the needs of individual patients at different stages during recovery is now laying such a foundation.

This book attempts to integrate a number of different elements which are prominent in rehabilitative medicine. Treatment approaches are presented in the context of clinical models, providing (where possible) a rationale for treatment, and linking therapy techniques to treatment results which have social and functional significance.

Part One attempts to define the problem of head injury, not only in terms of its size, but also in respect of its impact upon society and the family. A number of excellent research studies have been conducted which describe the 'burden' of head injury upon the family (Brooks et al., 1986) but no research study can ever convey the full impact of brain injury upon the social fabric of family life. The first chapter attempts to do this by outlining the different stages in the family's ability to gain awareness of the implications of brain injury. Reg Talbott is able to appreciate the nature and extent of the problem, both as co-founder and first director of the National Head Injuries Association in Great Britain. The emotional impact of this chapter is balanced by the epidemiological work of Dr John Bryden who has conducted a detailed study of head injury victims in selected Scottish health authorities, assessing both the incidence and prevalence of injury, and showing the accumulating number of 'lame brains' (London, 1967) who will require long-term care or supervision in the community.

Part Two attempts to provide a foundation for the practice of brain injury rehabilitation by suggesting **models of organization**. In 1980, the World Health Organization put forward a model of rehabilitation, but this simply divided the consequences of injury or disease into three levels: impairment, disability and handicap. This report did not attempt to provide an operational perspective that would integrate the diversity of individuals and disciplines who work with patients in a rehabilitation setting; neither did it attempt to define treatment goals in a way that directly linked the *goals* of treatment to the *practice* of treatment.

Chapter 3 by Eames and Wood looks at the structure and content of a head injury rehabilitation service, with particular reference to the types of patients that require treatment, the organization of therapy staff, and the goals of the rehabilitation programme. Chapters 4 and 5 go one step further in offering alternative perspectives for a rehabilitation service, with Eames recommending that specialist centres be established, capable of dealing with all aspects of brain injury and, in particular, the more serious management problems imposed by particular forms of behavioural disorder. An alternative approach is offered by Evans and Skidmore in Chapter 5. They describe the organization of rehabilitation in a community setting, when circumstances do not make it possible for the referral of brain-injured individuals to specialist centres. The value of these chapters is that they do not offer an 'either/or' alternative to rehabilitation but deal with some of the practical realities of providing treatment services under circumstances where the organization of health care may differ considerably.

Part Three considers some of the major ingredients of treatment methods in brain injury rehabilitation. Wood (Chapter 6) attempts to provide a foundation for organizing different aspects of treatment, based on a knowledge of brain injury and its recovery characteristics. In Chapter 7, Berrol deals with the management of physical disorders following brain injury, including methods of medication as well as different forms of physical medicine that will promote recovery and reduce disability and social handicap. Wilson, in Chapter 8, deals with the very important area of cognitive rehabilitation. There continues to be some debate about the clinical effectiveness and utility of cognitive rehabilitation procedures, but it is clear from recent follow-up studies of head-injured survivors that cognitive factors are more important than physical disability in helping a patient return to work or survive as an independent member of the community.

Training for community living has been a sadly neglected part of brain injury rehabilitation in the UK but has become more established in the USA where it is seen as an important stage in the continuum of rehabilitation. The chapter by Goll and Hawley (9) looks at the role of the transition living centre as a model for social rehabilitation, one which has proved clinically successful and extremely cost-effective in helping the most severely brain-injured individuals transfer from the clinic to the community. Finally, in Part Three, Eames looks at the 'risk-benefit considerations in drug treatment'. There is no doubt that many forms of medication prescribed for brain-injured patients (at any stage in their recovery, but especially during the early recovery period) can produce serious adverse consequences. Cognition may be blunted, slowing down the rate of recovery, or introducing an element of confusion which will exacerbate behaviour problems, and prejudice the outcome of the rehabilitation process.

Part Four deals specifically with the way treatment in rehabilitation is evaluated and the criteria of successful outcome determined. Evans (Chapter 11) presents an interesting set of data on long-term outcome of patients who have been provided with a comprehensive programme of rehabilitation therapy. This chapter is dedicated to the analysis of data from one specific rehabilitation centre. Chapter 12 by Haffey and Johnson provides an information system which looks at many of the elements contributing to rehabilitation outcome, advising on ways to judge their effectiveness. The content of this chapter is based upon the authors' experience conducting a comprehensive outcome study for a major rehabilitation organization in the USA.

In summary, therefore, two major problems in rehabilitation are addressed – 1. how to manage the individual patient and 2. the underlying organization of services. It is clear that a holistic approach is needed to the rehabilitation of patients with neurological disability. Wade (1987) suggests that it is easy to manage such disabled patients badly but 'probably impossible to do it perfectly'. Whilst this latter may be true it may be that any lesser aim will lead to distinctly lesser achievements.

Difficulties arise from the range of factors which need to be considered when organizing rehabilitation services. It is hoped that this book may offer some stimulus to professionals of all disciplines engaged in rehabilitation, encouraging a better understanding of the need to integrate the diverse elements of rehabilitation medicine, and directing them towards realistic treatment goals, using procedures which have their roots in clinical science, and are capable of objective evaluation.

RLW
PGE
1988

REFERENCES

Brooks, D.N., Campsie, L., Symington, C. *et al.*, (1986) The five year outcome of severe blunt head injury: a relatives view. *J. Neurol., Neurosurg. Psychiat.*, **49**, 764–70.

London, P.S. (1986) Some observations on the course of events after severe head injury. *Ann. R. Coll. Surg.*, **41**, 460–79.

Wade, D.T. (1987) Neurological rehabilitation. *Int. Disabil. Studies*, **9**, 45–47.

PART ONE

Understanding
the problem

1   The brain-injured person and the family

Reg Talbott

Head injury injures a family and for that family there are at least three crises following the injury:

1.1 THE FIRST CRISIS Announcment

The first crisis comes when the telephone rings, or the policeman calls, to say that a family member has been admitted to the local hospital and the doctors have requested immediate attendance by a close relative. On arrival the relative is presented with a life or death situation which may go on for hours or days, and the most common early complaint of relatives is that they are told nothing and can find no one to ask. These difficulties may be a result of a simple failure to understand on the part of the relatives (Thomsen, 1974) or as part of a much more fundamental process such as denial (Romano, 1974). The fact that relatives feel aggrieved after the communication they receive cannot be disputed. Whether or not it is a simple breakdown of communication or a failure to understand what is said, an absence of information can only make the situation worse for the very anxious relative.

Panting and Merry (1972) found that just over half of the relatives they interviewed said that supportive services had not been adequate and this was usually because doctors were thought to have supplied insufficient information. Such information was felt to be particularly lacking with regard to the patient's future prognosis and the difficulties which might be encountered in the future. Oddy's results (Oddy, Humphrey and Uttley, 1978) were very similar in that 40% of the relatives in his study had some criticism to make.

Not only are there problems of communication, there are also major problems of identification. Relatives are confronted by numerous people in uniforms, many of which are almost identical and others which give no indication of status or profession. The words 'neurosurgery', 'psychology' and 'therapy' rarely enter into the lives of ordinary people and yet they will be mentioned many times in the next 12 to 18 months. Everyone who works in this field will have been asked, 'What is neurosurgery?'; 'What does acute mean?'; 'What is rehabilitation?', and so on when the relatives have the courage to ask. Often they do not ask. In addition, relatives often ask 'Who is . . .?', because they have problems in distinguishing the different individuals involved in the patient's management.

The early hours are often remembered by relatives as some kind of obscure mystery play in which they attempt to come to terms with the early stages of family anxiety and grief. Surgeons and others dealing with the patient certainly have their own anxieties about presenting what they perceive to be the real picture to the relatives. Clinicians often feel that it is better to paint a bleak picture of the future so that any improvement can be recognized as an added bonus. Relatives very often complain about this portrayal afterwards, but are in no position to challenge it at the time.

Trauma is unlike many other medical situations in that the doctors have not met the patient before, and have had no prior communication with the relatives. Few other hospital situations result in the patient being unable to speak for days or weeks, with all the relevant clinical information obtained from specialized tests, observations and questioning of third parties. The doctor has not met the family before and even the most experienced clinician will find it hard in the early days to assess the strengths and capabilities of the relatives. He needs to know how much information or anxiety they can cope with while still continuing to function in their other daily activities.

On top of the difficulties of communication and identification, intensive care or intensive therapy units are an electronic nightmare to relatives entering for the first time. They do not generally want to know precisely what the equipment is for but they do want to know why it is necessary, and whether its very presence indicates that the outcome is likely to be very poor for their relative. After several hours of such anxiety, relatives find it very hard to believe that the patient will not wake up and immediately start to converse or somehow communicate. The popular view is that head injuries may result in brief coma and that after coma recovery is quick and complete. The entertainment and news media are largely to blame for this as the survivors of road accidents and other major catastrophes are often only media material for 24 hours until another story breaks. The long struggle for health is of much less media interest.

1.2 THE SECOND CRISIS

Hospital Transfers

family faced w/ trama actions

Days pass and relatives are often faced with a series of ward and hospital transfers. Again, questions often go unasked and therefore unanswered and painful journeys, both for the patient and the family, take place, introducing them to other hospitals, other consultants and other therapists. So the second crisis comes for many people when they realize that the patient is no longer likely to die in hospital but will have a prolonged period of limited recovery at the end of which the families still confidently expect perfection. Even with the best will in the world and open communication by therapists and others concerning handicap, few families can face the long-term prospects at this early stage. Indeed, families are well aware by this time that therapists have been actively working with the patient and they may see that the patient is starting to rouse from the coma; to a family member this may still presuppose complete recovery.

When asked about the situation at home and matters outside the hospital many relatives will indicate that they have totally ignored their responsibilities, other than to small children and elderly relatives. Often they have told their friends, employers, neighbours and others that the situation must take precedence. However, when asked how the patient is progressing, relatives lack the vocabulary to express their own difficulties or the progress of the patient. 'Getting on as well as can be expected', tends to be the most used phrase and this may have to satisfy both enquirer and relative for a considerable time. Very frequently however, friends drop away when they are not involved in the recovery process and are not being provided with the type of information that they normally expect to hear about friends in hospitals for other reasons. If psychological and behavioural abnormalities follow head injury, the spouses and close friends may try to distance themselves, forcing concerned parents to revert to an earlier form of parental role in which the parents themselves act as the supervisors and social agents in their child's life. Some friends, extended family members and school colleagues may be brought in to rehabilitation situations from time to time but this tends to be the exception rather than the rule. Other honourable exceptions include, for example, the family dog being pressed into service as a tangible reminder of days gone by and the solidarity of the family.

Once the patient begins to show signs of consciousness, the problems facing the family change and relatives now ask why the patient is so different, particularly in the case of those patients who have no broken bones, or scars or any other physical manifestations, and yet seem so totally different. Perhaps he is now a dazed and shattered figure with childish habits, limited awareness and poor physical shape, even after intense therapy. Family reorganization may begin at this stage with parents making decisions about their home, their employment and their job promotion. This reorganization can be very positive, yet it has a negative aspect: in a growing family where the patient is one of the children, siblings tend to be ignored, their interests put on one side. Indeed, in some cases they have become so discouraged that they leave home, often without any significant demur or acknowledgement by the parents. So often siblings hold very different views from the parents about the patient, both pre-accident and post-accident, and this can perhaps best be seen as a conflict between idolization on the part of the parents and stark reality as seen by other and younger persons.

Eventually, the father of an injured patient will resume his normal employment, although often he has to reduce his working hours and be at home more often and may decline opportunities for overtime, promotion and transfer. The mother may cease her full-time employ-ment or cut it to a minimum in order to resume the caring role she undertook very early after injury. Frequently patients are discharged from hospital prematurely at the insistence or request of relatives. All too often one hears relatives saying 'I can give more time to them at home if you train me and after all, what good is one hour of therapy a day when I can offer ten. Show me how to do it.' Indeed, 'Teach me', is a regular cry of relatives just prior to a request for an earlier discharge. Reasons families put forward for early discharge include:

1. travelling less to hospital
2. familiarity with surroundings at home
3. a shortage of money from lack of the patient's income
4. unexpected expenditure by the family
5. a recognition of the slowing down in the rate of recovery

1.3 THE THIRD CRISIS Discharge home.

It is at this point that another crisis will appear. Discharge home for medical and orthopaedic patients usually means a period of recovery and recuperation coupled with physical exercise and then a return to school, college or employment. The head-injured patient may be in no position to return to any of these and the family begins to fully realize that the return home marks the end of the time-limited intervention of hospital and rehabilitation unit. All the care previously shared by a hospital staff team now falls on one or two family members.

The first period at home may be one of euphoria, or of disillusionment. The travelling to and from hospital is no longer a chore but the amount of time devoted to the patient may distort every other family activity. Not only are there to be broken days but also broken nights, with periods of incontinence, disruptive behaviour and sometimes unaccountable lethargy. If the discharge has gone to plan, then the relatives will have been briefed on the situation with regard to physical and emotional needs, practical suggestions and help and arrangements being made for clinic visits and assessment. If, as in many cases, the discharge has been made prematurely, and at the insistence of family, then the picture of euphoria will be tinged with disappointment. Most relatives are unaware of the workings of a hospital which allow phenomena such as incontinence to be dealt with rapidly and dispassionately. For the relative, incontinence is a major problem that they may not have encountered before, except perhaps in child rearing. Naturally, relatives expect that the behaviour of the patient will change for the better when he returns to his home environment. Sadly, many of the expectations of the relatives will not be fulfilled and the burden of care will be a major task for the family from now on.

Siblings may feel antagonistic or alienated by the attention the patient receives, yet because they do not wish to create anxieties to add to their parents' worries, they now try to cope with their worries entirely on their own.

On the basis of Dr John Bryden's figures (Chapter 2), our patient is likely to be in his early twenties and the parents aged between 45 and 65 years. The patient is more likely to be male by a ratio of at least 3:1. Families have material and financial commitments that are based on normal assumptions, such as mortgages, life assurance etc. and ultimately the necessity of accepting life with only one major income whether it be from father or patient's wife, will result in financial stress in the years following rehabilitation.

1.4 HELPING THE FAMILY

Clinical services   *Finding support*

Where does the support come from? Many hospital social workers are skilled in work with children and with the elderly. However, with head injuries forming only a relatively small number of hospital patients and approximately one in eight hundred of the population (Bryden, 1986), the difficulties facing patient and family may not be fully understood unless the social worker is attached to a neurosurgery or accident and emergency unit on a permanent or regular basis. The social worker should be able to deal with the minefield of social welfare benefits. Occupational therapists, together with physiotherapists will have played a vital role in the treatment of the patient and may have been able to carry out appropriate discharge planning, including arranging for appropriate assistance by providing equipment and adaptations to the home property. Many social services departments however, are limited in such resources and there may be a lengthy period of negotiation between social service departments, housing departments and the owner of the property.

Vocational rehabilitation

Whilst rehabilitation centres may have assessed the abilities of the patient and made suggestions through the various specialized rehabilitation staff as to appropriate re-employment, millions of able-bodied unemployed people compete with the disabled employee and he has a reduced chance of finding a satisfying form of employment. Additionally, the head-injured patient will have been out of work for many months and modern industry and technology will have passed him by. Training and re-training schemes are available for handicapped people, but the mixture of physical and cognitive problems faced by the head-injured person will make him less able to train and come to terms with new techniques and facilities. Even if the employer is able to find a situation in which the employee can be accommodated it may be less satisfying, less well-paid and have less status than the original post. The employer may not wish to place the employee in a situation which risks the lives and livelihoods of others.

1.5 LATE PROBLEMS

Safety judgement

If the ex-patient cannot return to work, how far can he be trusted to do things for himself and look after himself even in the family home? Forgetting to turn off the gas tap, water tap or the electric cooker may be something that we all do from time to time, but when this happens daily, it is expensive and can result in other serious consequences which may affect, and have to be remedied by other people. Flooded bathrooms and kitchens may be the price that a family has to pay for the restoration of dignity to the patient, and burnt saucepans and spoilt food may pre-determine the ex-patient's ability to provide meals again for himself.

Driving

Learning to drive and having responsibility for the safety of a vehicle may be only half the problem encountered by the relatives faced with someone who might be utterly lost when only 20 miles from the family home. In Britain the Department of Transport seems to be inconsistent in its handling of head-injured patients. Some have been forbidden to drive on medical advice whilst others have resumed their driving only to find that regulations prevent them from continuing. A proper assessment by the appropriate authorities is necessary here so that the regulations can be fully understood by all concerned and, if necessary, representations made to the Department by those in charge of the case.

Education

Education, and particularly re-education, are vital aspects of recovery after head injury. A small but increasing number of hospitals and rehabilitation centres are involving educational therapists and teachers in this work, alongside psychologists and the other therapists. Everyone has an educational role in some form or other but formalized education for most people means returning to school, further education or higher education. Many patients have physical problems which prevent them from undertaking the tasks that they did previously; computers and other communication aids may help patients compensate for these deficits. Literacy and numeracy tutors can be found in the community through the schemes that have been operating for many years, and in some colleges of further education there are courses which, although filled exclusively with handicapped people, offer opportunities for testing oneself against others. Even in higher education, ex-patients have returned to universities and polytechnics with staff making appropriate adjustments; the outcome has not always been a satisfactory one, however, with patients failing examinations after being led to believe that they will be successful by an overdose of confidence-boosting, help and guidance.

Marital problems

Sadly, many patients have little to offer to their marriage after head injury, and changed sexual abilities and disabilities may give rise to changed relationships. In one instance, well known to me, the ex-patient returned home to his slightly injured wife and found that he could not recall ever marrying the woman and did not realize that he was the father of the child of the home. She has continued to look after him, accepting her legal and moral responsibilities, but there is clearly a gulf between them which can never be fully bridged by any kind of external intervention. Some researchers have indicated that marriage and family relationships may be tested to the extreme and still survive whilst others believe that the divorce rate amongst head-injured people and their spouse is higher than average. The latter seems much more likely: relatives and others work hard to maintain relationships, but a breaking point for some will come later rather than sooner.

1.6 HEADWAY

For all the reasons stated above and others, Headway, the National Head Injuries Association in the UK was formed in 1979 to help families come to terms with their difficulties and assist professionals in their work with such families. The need for this organization, and for kindred organizations in the United States and Australia, is borne out by their growth over the last 9 years. At the time of writing, Headway has over 70 active self-help and support groups in the UK with many others planned.

The original thinking of the founders of Headway was that much work could be done with families in small groups at the time of the expressed need. This does not always occur during the first few days after the accident, but becomes more important once family stresses reach crisis points, when opinions other than those held by doctors and therapists can be brought to bear on the problem. Solutions laboriously worked out by other families might be just the answer that a new family is looking for. Headway also found that the lack of understanding of the problem extended further than the families with injured relatives, to the general public. Thus, many media oppor-tunities have been taken advantage of. This has inevitably rebounded on the organization at times, producing many more enquiries than expected but the message seems to be getting home. In addition, publications and booklets have been produced by the organization, written generally by professional workers*. Although these were targeted initially at the families asking for help and basic information,

* Headway publications are available from: National Head Injuries Association, 200 Mansfield Road, Nottingham, NG1 3HX.

thousands of these have now been freely distributed to families or bought by younger or less experienced professional workers coming into this particular field.

The grass roots

In 1984 Gillian Talbott undertook a study of the members of Headway groups (Talbott, 1984). Questionnaires were sent out to the coveners of the then 44 groups and the replies came from 132 members. This concerned the demographic features of the population (age, occupation etc.), severity of injury and knowledge and expectations of Headway.

The relationship of the patient to the carer was interesting, 89 parents and 33 husbands or wives answered the questionnaire, a 3:1 ratio of parents to spouses (Table 1.1). The patients were mainly young people and the majority required family support. Only eight of the individuals surveyed lived alone whilst 96 lived with 1–6 other people in a family. Of the 132 patients sampled at the time of the study, 107 were by then at home.

The figures produced by Bryden (1986), concerning the age of the patient at the time of administration to hospital, were supported by this study (see Table 1.2).

Table 1.3 shows that a large number of patients in the groups were involved in vehicle accidents especially with motor cars, contrary to a popular belief that head injuries are generally associated with young motorcyclists. Twenty one people had a coma of up to 1 week, 40 people up to 4 weeks and 43 people up to 3 months. Ninety participants reported patients with memory problems exceeding 6 months duration. The vast majority of patients returned home within 6 months but others had not returned home 2 years after the accident. One was returned home without a period of in-patient admission to the hospital – an unusual situation.

The number of patients finding Headway through various sources resulted directly in a change in the approach to publicity. The

Table 1.1. Position of patient within the family

Mother	Father	Spouse	Children				Other	Independent	Total
			1st	2nd	3rd	4th			
7	26	5	38	28	12	3	11	2	132/132

Table 1.2. Ages of patients at time of admission to hospital

Age (years)	Number of patients
0–10	5
10–15	10
16–20	37
21–25	28
26–30	16
31–40	17
41–50	13
50–60	3
60+	3
Total	132

Table 1.3. Causes of injury resulting in brain damage

Cause of injury	Number of patients
Car	54
Motorcycle	20
Cycle	5
Hit by vehicle	15
Assault	3
Industrial accident	5
Sport	4
Home	9
Other	17
Total	132

Table 1.4 Sources of referral to Headway

Source	Number of referrals
Doctor	10
Physiotherapist	6
Occupational therapist	8
Psychologist	3
Speech therapist	15
Social worker	38
Nurse	5
Another family	11
Another patient	1
Media	39
Existing group	3
DRO	1
MIND	2

expectations of the local group members conformed closely to those which the founders had predicted. They are summarized as follows:

1. Moral support, sharing problems with others with the same experiences, discussion and companionship;
2. Promoting educational talks, giving advice on rehabilitation, facilities etc;
3. Helping to alleviate feelings of isolation and loneliness by organizing social activities for patients and families;
4. Helping patients to come to terms with the situation by meeting others;
5. Informal contact with the professionals;
6. Acting as a local publicity medium and pressure group;
7. Providing a telephone link;
8. Helping with legal advice, welfare rights and contact with rehabilitation facilities;
9. Helping with problems of communication and frustration due to speech problems;
10. Providing long-term support and contact for families.

When respondents were asked about their expectations of Headway nationally, rather than locally, the findings were as follows:

1. Providing literature, publicity; influencing national policy on provision for the brain-injured;
2. Keeping local groups informed of new developments and research, such as new treatments, benefits and technical developments;
3. Coordinating activities of the groups;
4. Providing a centralized information and advice service covering the range of questions asked by families;
5. Acting as a public voice at a national level, as a pressure group; lobbying Members of Parliament;
6. Instigating research, particularly into long-term needs;
7. Providing training for families;
8. Starting more groups;
9. Providing residential care, hostels, sheltered housing and pressing for special units within the National Health Service.

Seventy six of those surveyed suggested that they did not particularly need Headway to provide rented and supervised accommodation, 34 requested this facility and another 19 asked for more information about it. Similarly, 79 indicated that they would not be interested in buying a property supervised by Headway, 38 suggested they would and 20 requested more information.

The information from the questionnaire confirmed many of the needs of which the original founders of Headway had been aware. It demonstrated the categories of patients by age groups, type of accident, forms of care and gave members the opportunity (anonymously) to express their expectations. Obviously, those coming to a Headway group or merely being in contact, have quite definite ideas of what they expect to gain from belonging to a network of support groups which are part of a national organization, and these expectations are now a focus of Headway. Robinson and Robinson (1979) say:

> The good groups help newcomers, old members and often professionals and the general public as well, to overcome the practical problems associated with their particular illness, disability or problem.

In the long-term, therefore, Headway's plans include a range of appropriate means of care. Initially, two day centres were established, the first in Gloucester and the second in Basingstoke, to provide for the needs of patients after leaving hospital. Both centres developed after local groups had been in operation for some years and the needs of the patients and families, past and present, were analysed. Whilst providing opportunities for learning to budget, cook, clean and communicate, other individual projects arose to enable people to prepare themselves for independence or perhaps further education. Over 120 ex-patients have now passed through the Gloucester Day Centre operated by Headway Cotswold, and the daily costs have been so little that at least another six day centres are likely to be opened in the UK before the summer of 1988. Even where there is no prospect of a patient returning to education or employment the fact that a member is in a safe environment for several days each week provides respite for the harassed family at home and an opportunity to review their position and future needs.

Headway is now working with other charities and voluntary organizations. Plans are in hand for the first joint venture with the Leonard Cheshire Foundation and a rehabilitation home will be opened in Stockport, probably during 1989. The high capital cost of such premises and the substantial running costs will be negotiated between the organizations and will ensure maximum benefit being derived from the input of each agency.

Organization of Headway

Headway acts as an umbrella over individual groups, allowing each to be autonomous and function according to the needs of the local members. This is dictated partly by the way it was originally started (whether by patients, families or professionals) and partly by the geographic location of hospitals and the areas from which patients are drawn. Within an urban area it is much easier to meet other families who have been through the same major accident hospital than it is to meet such people in areas such as the Scottish Highlands, North Yorkshire Moors, Southern Ireland or even Australia.

At a recent meeting of a local Headway group in the south east of England the members tried to analyse the benefit of belonging to the group; many useful comments and statements were made. One thing which came to light over and over again is that love has a large part to play in the recovery of the head-injured person. Not just loving the person concerned, but also loving everyone involved. The support of family and friends was said to be essential and a sense of humour is a great help as well!

Most people present at that meeting felt that they benefited from being involved with Headway. Everyone was prepared to try and help anyone who is unfortunate enough to find themselves in similar circumstances. They said that if they could reach the people who need this type of support soon after the injury occurs, then perhaps they could make them feel less isolated than they themselves had felt.

A speaker at Headway, Southampton, said recovery from head injury is a learning process and not a healing process, and that any learning is inevitably individual. It is necessary to remember what kind of personality the injured person had before the accident. Jennett (1972) noted that even though the patient may have made a satisfactory recovery and good social adjustment, his spouse may avow that he is not the man she married. Since this is a relatively new, 20th century syndrome, the story is only now becoming apparent and the future will show the needs of patients as they and their families grow older, towards the end of this century.

REFERENCES

Bryden, J. (1986) Unpublished epidemiological study of populations in the west of Scotland with particular reference to head injury.

Jennett, B. (1972) Late Effects of Head Injuries (Scientific Foundations of Neurology) Heinemann, London.

Oddy, M., Humphrey, M.E. and Uttley, D. (1978) Subjective Impairment of Social Recovery after Closed Head Injury. J. Neurol., Neurosurg. Psychiat., 41, 611–16.

Panting, A. and Merry, P. (1972) The Long-term Rehabilitation of Severe Head Injuries with Particular Reference to the Need for Social and Medical Support for the Patient's Family. Rehabilitation, 38, 33–7.

Robinson, D. and Robinson, Y. (1979) *From Self-help to Health*, Concord Books, London.

Romano, M.D. (1974) Family Response to Traumatic Head Injury. *Scand. J. Rehabil. Med.*, **6**, 1–4.

Talbott, G. (1984) *Headway – An Assessment of a Self-help and Support Group for Families of Head Injured Patients*, Dissertation for University of Nottingham.

Thomsen, I.V. (1974) The Patient with Severe Head Injury and His Family. *Scand. J. Rehabil. Med.*, **6**, 180–83.

2

How many head-injured? The epidemiology of post head injury disability

John Bryden

The word 'epidemiology' is rather a mouthful, but it is a very necessary and helpful discipline. Statistics on their own may be misleading; epidemiology gives health statistics real perspective in terms of time and place. The evidence presented in this chapter is drawn mainly from the work of the Scottish Head Injury Management Study (SHIMS) funded by the Medical Research Council and the Scottish Chief Scientist's Office, and led by Jennett and Teasdale. The author was fortunate to work with this study for 3 years.

Some basic definitions are required in the interpretation of the data which follow. The definition of the **incidence** of a condition is the number of new cases of the condition arising in a given population in a given period of time, for example, the number of newly disabled joining the total pool of all disabled over the course of a year. The definition of the related measure, **prevalence**, is the total number of people suffering from the condition in a given population at a given point in time, for example, the number in the total pool of those who are disabled at present.

2.1 HEAD INJURIES SEEN IN HOSPITAL

There are many definitions of 'head injury'. In some areas, mainly urban ones, a useful definition is 'a blow on the head severe enough for the victim to seek hospital advice or care'. In more rural areas this might need to be altered to '**medical** advice or care'. In the Scottish study, however, the 'attendance at hospital' definition was used, and it has to be recognized that this does lead to a degree of under-estimation of very minor injuries, and of course it omits those who are killed at the site of the accident and therefore do not reach hospital care.

In order to make full sense of the data, it is necessary to have an understanding of the pattern of head injury care in most parts of Britain (and, indeed, Europe). In the first instance, injured patients make their way, by ambulance or otherwise, to an accident and emergency department at a local hospital. Here, each patient is assessed, and investigated by X-rays and routine laboratory tests. Most patients are fit to be discharged home at this stage, but some are admitted overnight for observation for early recognition of possible complications, and are discharged home within 48 hours.

There is a small proportion whose condition causes some particular concern, possibly prompted by specific local or national advisory guidelines (*Brit. Med. J.*, 1984). Such patients are transferred to the regional neurosurgical service, where specialized skilled assessment and neurological investigations are available. According to the findings, the patient may then return to the referring hospital, or may stay until neurosurgical or other special treatment is completed. As recovery proceeds, rehabilitation therapies are begun at the regional service, but most patients are returned to the referring hospital quite quickly, for further care until they are ready for discharge home.

This model of care has the advantage of concentrating scarce high-technology skills, and making them equally available to all of the regional population. It promotes a fast turnover of patients in the regional beds, and ensures that space is available for new referrals. However, it does mean that patients and their families are subjected to changes of care environment, and that most rehabilitation is under-taken in a setting (i.e. the local hospital) where experience is limited because only small numbers of head-injured patients are seen.

2.2 HOW MANY HEAD INJURIES HAPPEN?

How many head injured are there? Our expectations might be, on the one hand, increased by newspaper headlines and television news items or, on the other hand, decreased by the relative invisibility of disabled people in our society. Detailed studies are needed to paint the true picture. If a study is to be reliable, it must be conducted within clearly defined geographical boundaries, and SHIMS has been lucky in this respect. The West of Scotland Regional Institute of Neurological Sciences serves a defined catchment area of 2.7 million people, distributed between centralized urban, country town, village, and even isolated rural settings. There are both industry and gross unemployment, affluence and social disadvantage. It is argued that these characteristics allow the study to be taken as a representative guide to the frequency and pattern of head injuries in the country as a whole.

The Scottish studies have shown that attendance at an accident department because of head injury has an incidence of one in fifty of the total population in each year (Strang et al., 1978). This amounts to about 11% of the new work-load in these units. Over 75% were able to return home without admission.

On initial survey of Scotland in 1974, 300 people per 100 000 of the population were admitted each year because of head injury (Jennett and Macmillan, 1981). However, the incidence varies according to the availability of local care facilities (Brit. Med. J., 1984) and the cultural patterns of accidents. In England and Wales at that time, the overall figure was 270, and in some parts of the United States it may be much lower.

The number of patients undergoing neurosurgical treatment also varies very considerably, and depends on the availability of resources, and on local policies (Brit. Med. J., 1984; Jennett and Macmillan, 1981; Bryden and Jennett, 1983). In Merseyside only 1% of head injury admissions were admitted to neurosurgical units, in most of Scotland the figure was about 5%, but in Teeside it was 25%. In Lothian and south-east Scotland, which have access to a minor and major head injury ward in Edinburgh, 35% of head injury admissions go to that unit.

There is a strong case for the setting of targets to provide regional neurosurgical facilities for the head injured in order to optimize outcome. This was well argued during a multidisciplinary seminar organized by the Department of Health and Social Security in Harrogate in 1983, and made public in several resulting papers (Bryden and Jennett, 1983; Lewis, 1983), and in the nationally recommended guidelines (Brit. Med. J., 1984). A very recent publication (Brocklehurst et al., 1987) reports on the implementation of these guidelines in practice, and supports the earlier view that at least ten neurosurgical head injury beds are required for the effective management of the head-injured for each one million of the population.

2.3 SOCIAL ASPECTS OF HEAD INJURY

What sorts of people suffer head injury, and in what ways? The answers vary from study to study. Table 2.1 summarizes the findings of the Scottish study with reference to the effects of the degree of severity.

Deaths

Mortality data always have to be treated with statistical caution. The quality of the information is only as good as the quality of the certification. Deaths following head injury may occur at the scene of the accident, *en route* to hospital, in the primary hospital, *en route* to neurosurgical care, in the regional unit, in long-term care settings, or in the home. The numbers and relative proportions of deaths in these various places are affected by many aspects of health promotion and accident prevention.

It is apparent from Table 2.1 that what might be called the 'macho image' (devil-may-care attitudes, alcohol, and violence) figures prominently in the causation of head injury. Can educational policies be effective in changing this, or is legislative action the only way? Police action on drink and driving, and the 1983 UK seat belt legislation, have certainly produced change (Rutherford *et al.*, 1985). Jennett and Carlin (1978) showed, from autopsies of those dying early after head injury, that some deaths might have been preventable by more active first-aid measures. Gentleman and Jennett (1981), Price and Murray (1972) and Graham *et al.* (1978) have demonstrated both some causes and the effects of cerebral hypoxia and ischaemia. The head injury guidelines previously mentioned were introduced in order to try to optimize National Health Service care of the head-injured. All of these factors have influenced mortality from head injury in the UK.

The falling mortality rate has not necessarily reduced either the work-load of the health services or the incidence of new morbidity. For example, there is some evidence that the wearing of seat belts has shifted the pattern of severity of injuries in the following ways: from major and minor injury to no injury; from major injury to minor injury; and from death to survival with major injury. Reviews by the Department of Health and Social Security before and after the introduction of seat belt legislation, and also the work continuing in Glasgow, appear to support this view (Registrar General for Scotland, 1980; Rutherford *et al.*, 1985; Murray, 1987).

Table 2.1 Severity of head injuries and changing causes[a]

	Only seen in A and E[b] sent home (%)	Needed 'overnight' in PSW[c] (%)	Merited transfer to NSU[d] (%)	'Severe' injuries (%)	Deaths (%)
Road accidents	13	34	38	58	56
Assaults	23	20	11	7	7
Alcoholic falls	7	12	19	16	29
Work (not road)	12	7	9	7	4
Sample cases	2735	1181	424	1000	476

[a]   From the Scottish Head Injury Management Study
[b] A and E   ·Accident and emergency departments
[c] PSW   Primary surgical wards
[d] NSU   Neurosurgical unit

After head injury

This book is principally about the problems of the head-injured when they have returned to the community. So far this chapter has simply outlined the incidence of head injury: each year, for every million of the population, 20 000 will attend an accident department; 3 000 will be admitted to a local hospital; 200 will be transferred for neurosurgical investigation or treatment. But what happens then? About 20 of the 200 transferred will die, either shortly or (in a few cases) after some months in a 'persistent vegetative state'. About 160 of the 200 will make a reasonable recovery. Twenty new people per million of population per year will be left with considerable disability, despite the best of treatment and care.

This latter figure was calculated from the SHIMS data in the early 1980s, and it is interesting that it corresponds closely with P.S. London's calculation in 1967 (London, 1967). What does this incidence of new disability mean to society as a whole? It has to be remembered that the average age of injury is in the twenties, and that the expectation of life for those so disabled appears to be normal. Some will have 50 to 60 years of disability ahead of them.

In order to plan adequate provision for these disabled individuals, one needs to know not only the incidence of new cases in each year, but also the prevalence of continuing disability. The former can be measured from neurosurgical units; assessment of the latter is much more difficult. It is possible to make actuarial calculations based on the age structure of those sustaining and surviving disabling head injury in a given year, assuming an average expectation of life. From the Glasgow data, experimental calculations of this sort suggest a prevalence of about 35 000 people disabled from head injury in the UK. Table 2.6 emphasizes, however, the problems of extrapolation. Perhaps the greatest errors arise from varying professional and public concepts of disability and handicap. These predictions have been arrived at by multiplying the rates found in the various studies to give a predicted rate for the whole of the UK. As the Strathclyde studies have been based on total populations, and three different types of populations, each with the very high response rate of 97% of households, it is argued that their mid-point estimate of one per thousand population is probably the most likely figure.

It seemed a more accurate approach, however, to undertake a community study to measure the prevalence of head injury disability more directly in British society. If resources are to be directed towards these problems, they must first be properly quantified.

Recent articles, and also reports by a coordinating group funded by the Medical Research Council (MRC,1982) and by a working party of the Royal College of Physicians (1986), have made strong recommendations for the development of new tailor-made services for head injury rehabilitation. Given the current finite boundaries for health and social service finance, such developments would have to take place at the expense of some other therapeutic activity. To justify such reallocation of resources, an accurate assessment of the size and economic impact of the problems is essential.

2.4 THE SCOTTISH STUDY OF PREVALENCE OF HEAD INJURY DISABILITY

Method

Community disability prevalence studies are notoriously difficult; each depends on someone's personal concept of disability and handicap. Amelia Harris' well known study (1971) used Office of Population and Census Surveys (OPCS) interviewing techniques. Knight and Warren (1978) reviewed the wide range of studies carried out by social service departments in England in the wake of the *Chronically Sick and Disabled Persons Act*, and of the 154 studies available they classed only

51 'good or excellent' as far as their survey techniques were concerned. Despite varying techniques, all of these studies suggest a community prevalence of disability (from all causes) of between 5 and 10% of the total population.

Strathclyde region in Scotland has a population of about 2.4 million, and without doubt the highest levels of multiple social deprivation in the United Kingdom. Its social work department has organized a 'rolling census' technique for the identification of people living in the community with long-term disability (by which is meant those who are disabled or handicapped in their own or their families' eyes). The regional council first delineates communities of 50 000 to 90 000 people, and then detailed discussions are held between each appropriate district council and the relevant health board, local community leaders and organizations, church leaders and so on. Financed by the Manpower Services Commission, large teams of research interviewers are hired locally. The teams are given 6 weeks of intensive training, in both interview techniques and more general aspects of disability, by relevant health professionals. All dwellings on the region's computer listing of rateable properties are visited (and in practice more than 95% of occupied households were surveyed in the study). The interviewers ask: 'Is there anyone living here whose every-day life is affected by illness, disability or injury, either physical or mental, or by problems due to age (e.g. arthritis, rheumatism or heart trouble), injury, or defect of sight, hearing or mobility?' If the answer is 'yes', the interviewers return later, hopefully with at least one further member of the household present, and complete a detailed question-naire.

The present study of head injury disability has 'piggy-backed' on this wider census, and in three zones has added to the questionnaire some simple questions designed to show whether any disability was the result of head injury. Irvine New Town in Ayrshire, with the much older adjoining Burghs of Ardrossan, Saltcoats and Stevenston, formed one zone, and the whole of Dumbarton district, and the Glasgow post-war development area known as Easterhouse, were the other two. Together the three zones comprise a population of 260 000, with a broad mixture of community types.

Findings

In each of the three studies, the overall disability rates from all causes were between 6 and 9% (Table 2.2). Of course, these studies measure disability – or 'handicap' or 'impairment' – as seen through the eyes of the community and lay enumerators. Many health professionals may

Table 2.2 Strathclyde sick and disabled persons project

	Study population (from 1981 census)	Identified	Disabled (%)	Staff	Cost (thousand pounds)
Dumbarton	76 937	4723	6.1	84	336
Easterhouse	80 701	5431	6.7	82	280
Irvine	91 279	7738	8.5	82	280

Table 2.3 Studies of community prevalence of disability

Date	Author	Community	Disabled (%)
1966	Skinner	Lambeth	4.4
1966/67	Bennett	Tower Hamlets	8.0
1968/69	Lowther	Exeter/Edinburgh	4.0
1968/69	Harris	UK	7.8 (of adults)
1974	Knight and Warren	Social work departments (a) Sample studies (b) Total household studies	15–31 9–18
1981 et seq.	Waldman	Strathclyde	6–10

Table 2.4 Rates standardized towards mean of disability (Pick up rates)

	Rates per 100 000	Standardized towards mean
Dumbarton	51	66
Easterhouse	86	101
Greater Irvine	123	114

have different concepts and definitions for these, but there is some movement towards agreed standards, in particular the international classification of the World Health Organization, 1980. Nevertheless, Table 2.3 shows that the Scottish rates are comparable to those from other UK studies, and it is therefore reasonable to argue that the head injury disability rates reported to these interviewers can be taken as valid for the UK as a whole. These are standardized for age, and then shown as mean general disability rates, in Table 2.4.

There is no obvious reason for the differences in prevalence between

Table 2.5 Community disease prevalence per 100 000

	Amelia Harris	Dumbarton	Easterhouse	Irvine
Multiple sclerosis	44*	65	35	57
Post polio	69*	59	41	70
Post head injury	22*	51*	86*	123*

* Age standardized

the three zones. Head injury incidence rates show a relationship with social disadvantage and lower socio-economic status, and from this one would expect the Easterhouse rate to be higher. It may be that the Dumbarton district community has a stricter concept of disability. Table 2.5 presents head injury disability rates in a 'league table' with other chronic disabling conditions, with surprising results. Perhaps public awareness is out of touch with how common the problem is.

Implications

The findings show that the annual flow (incidence) of two new patients per 100 000 of the population leads to a pool (prevalence) of about 100 people disabled by head injury for every 100 000. This suggests a total of about 55 000 such people in the UK (Table 2.6).

The average Health District (a quarter of a million population) will have some 250 people with lasting disability from head injury, and it has to be remembered that this means 250 disabled families. A particularly illuminating translation of these figures is that each general practitioner will have, on average, two such patients on his or her list. It may be that better coordination of community rehabilitation

Table 2.6 Predictions of post head injury disability prevalence

Study date	Source	Estimated disabled in UK
1968/69	Amelia Harris	12 000
1974–1981	SHIMS actuarial predictions	36 000
1974–1981	Scottish head injury discharge predictions	80 000
1982	Current study	
	Dumbarton	30 000
	Easterhouse	50 000
	Irvine	70 000

resources will lessen the amount of handicap associated with this disability, and studies are in progress to examine this possibility prospectively (Brooks *et al.*, 1986).

ACKNOWLEDGEMENTS

The author expresses his thanks to the wide group of researchers, medical records officers, secretaries and others, from whose work this chapter has been drawn.

REFERENCES

Brit. Med. J., **288**, 983–85 (1984). Guidelines for initial management after head injury in adults.

Brocklehurst, G., Gooding, M. and James, G. (1987) Comprehensive care for patients with head injuries. *Brit. Med. J.*, **294**, 345–47.

Brooks, D.N., Campsie, L.M., Beattie, A. *et al.* (1986) Head injury and the rehabilitation professions in the West of Scotland. *Health Bulletin (Edinburgh)*, **44** (2), 110–17.

Bryden, J. and Jennett, B. (1983) Neurosurgical resources and transfer policies for head injuries. *Brit. Med. J.*, **286**, 1791–93.

Gentleman, D. and Jennett, B. (1981) Hazards of inter-hospital transfer of comatose head-injured patients. *Lancet*, **ii**, 853–58.

Graham, D.I., Adams, J.H. and Doyle, D. (1978) Ischaemic brain damage in fatal non-missile head injuries. *J. Neurol. Sci.*, **39**, 213–34.

Harris, A. (1971) *Handicap and impairment in Great Britain*, OPCS, HMSO, London.

Jennett, B. and Carlin, J. (1978) Preventable mortality and morbidity after head injury. *Injury*, **10**, 31–39.

Jennett, B. and Macmillan, R. (1981) Epidemiology of head injury. *Brit. Med. J.*, **282**, 101–4.

Knight, R. and Warren, M. (1978) *Physically disabled people living at home: a study of numbers in need*, HMSO, London.

Lewis, A.F. (1983) *The management of acute head injury. Harrogate Seminar Report No 8*, HMSO and DHSS.

London, P.S. (1967) Some observations on the course of events after severe injury of the head. *Ann. R. Coll. Surg. Eng.*, **41**, 460–79.

Murray, S. (1987) *SHIMS – personal communication.*

MRC Coordinating Group Report (1982) Research aspects of rehabilitation after acute brain damage in adults. *Lancet*, **ii**, 1034–36.

Price, D.J.E. and Murray, A. (1972) Influence of hypoxia and hypotension on recovery from head injury. *Injury*, **2**, 218–24.

Registrar General for Scotland (1980) *Annual Report*, HMSO, Edinburgh.

Royal College of Physicians (1986) Physical disability in 1986 and beyond. *J. R. Coll. Phys.*, **20** (3), 20–21.

Rutherford, W.H., Greenfield, A., Hayes, H.R.M. and Nelson, J.K. (1985) *The Medical Effects of Seat Belt Legislation in the United Kingdom*, HMSO, London.

Strang, I., Macmillan, R. and Jennett, B. (1978) Scottish Head Injury Management Study: head injuries in accident and emergency departments in Scottish hospitals. *Injury*, **10**, 154–59.

World Health Organization (1980) *International Classification of Impairments, Disabilities and Handicaps: a Manual of Classification Relating to the Consequences of Disease*, WHO, Geneva.

PART TWO

Models of organization

3 The structure and content of a head injury rehabilitation service

Peter Eames
and Rodger Ll. Wood

In the last decade, studies of the nature of cognitive, affective, behavioural and personality deficits after head injury have increased rapidly, and interest has grown in the more difficult questions of what to do about these deficits. Just as importantly, the problems and needs of families have been taken increasingly seriously (Brooks, 1984; Brooks *et al.*, 1986). Professionals involved in the study and rehabilitation of the effects of head injury have learned an enormous amount from the promptings, questions and insights of families, and still have much more to learn.

Unfortunately, these insights have not yet reached a wide audience. In the UK, and to a lesser extent in the USA, rehabilitation centres continue to approach the head-injured as though physical disorders and rather primitive levels of activities of daily living were the only necessary targets of treatment. In the UK particularly, an atmosphere of retrenchment has pervaded the National Health Service for some years, leading to a dwindling of what little imaginative rehabilitation of the head-injured there has been. In the USA, head injury rehabilitation has become a 'growth industry', but the growth of private facilities has outstripped that of evaluation of treatment methods.

Unfortunate though this is, the present position does have some advantages. The growing pressure from both professionals and the public (spearheaded by Headway in the UK, and the National Head Injuries Foundation in the USA), and increasing availability of information about the numbers involved (Bryden, 1985 and Chapter 2 of this book; Royal College of Physicians, 1986), the economic impacts (Bryden, 1985), and the achievements which can be made (Berrol *et al.*, 1982; Eames and Wood, 1985b), are producing a climate in which new facilities and resources for head injury rehabilitation are certainly going to be developed.

What seems particularly important, therefore, is to ensure that what is developed is not only appropriate, but the best that can be designed, taking into account all of the experience and research findings of the last decade. As well as increasing our understanding of the problems, these findings have presented us with an implicit message: the span of deficits produced by diffuse head injury is very wide, and their rehabilitation demands the skills of an equally wide range of professional disciplines; thus, it is clear that, in seeking the best solutions to the problems of rehabilitation, we must cast our nets as widely as possible in the waters of human knowledge. This will amount to an extension of the present interdisciplinary approach to rehabilitation.

It is the purpose of this chapter to consider not only what is already known about the needs of a comprehensive rehabilitation service for the head-injured, but also fields which have not yet been fully explored in the search for the best that can be achieved.

3.1 THE DESIGN OF REHABILITATION: TERMS IN THE EQUATION

The effects of head injury

The patterns of damage to the brain produced by head injury have been described many times in the recent literature of the subject (e.g. Wood and Eames, 1981; Teasdale and Mendelow, 1984), and need not be reviewed at any length here. It is worth restating, however, that trauma to the head produces a combination of localized damage (from depressed or comminuted fracture, surface contusion, or intracranial haemorrhage) and scattered microscopic damage (from shearing and centrifugal pressure forces) in the brain. As a result there is likely to be interference with both localized specific brain functions, and the diffused modulatory functions (arousal, attention, drive). Moreover, *all* brain functions are likely to be affected by the reduction in speed of processing which results from a scattered loss of nerve fibres.

Effects on brain functions

Everything which we experience, know, think, plan, feel, will and do, is achieved through, and depends upon, brain functions. The rest of the body merely provides for the brain's needs or serves the brain's commands. As a result of the complex and diffuse damage of this organ and its comprehensive functions, there is a need for a rehabilitative effort in the wide range of functional areas in the following list.

Physical
Communication
Activities of daily living
   basic
   domestic
   community
Social skills
Cognitive

Behavioural
Emotional
Sexual
Medical/psychiatric
Family
Occupational
Recreational

Many of these have only recently been recognized as areas of specific need, and techniques of rehabilitation are actively being explored and researched around the world. Even in the more established areas (physical and communication therapies, for example) it has become apparent that there is much to be learned about suitable techniques (including the question of whether they actually have any effect). In particular, the close cooperation of different disciplines, applying different therapies to the same individual at the same time, is achieving results quite unexpectedly superior to those of more traditional approaches.

As a group, the severely head-injured often behave in unpredictable, unpleasant and even frightening ways. This often makes them rather unpopular with treatment staff. This is greatly magnified when they are mixed in with other groups of patients, because the contrast is highlighted. Increasing experience of dealing with the head-injured as a separate group, however, is showing that it becomes easy for the treaters to recognize and derive satisfaction from the progress that can be achieved, and to accept the patients as a norm. Comparisons with other types of patients are not immediately available, and staff do not have to worry about the unsettling and sometimes dangerous effects of the head-injured on others.

Cognitive, behavioural and family issues cut across the whole spectrum of physical and functional disorders after head injury, yet few therapists have training or experience in these areas. Understanding and expertise can, however, be developed by fostering much closer working relationships and interaction between different disciplines. This also serves as effective protection against manipulation by patients and their families, and reduces the latter's chance of misunderstanding information given them about the patient's condition.

Severity of injury

It is customary to classify the severity of injury in terms of the duration of coma or post-traumatic amnesia (PTA) (Russell and Smith, 1961; Teasdale and Jennett, 1974). However, there are problems with this method when it comes to rehabilitation. Whilst these measures do seem to correlate well on the whole with the degree of diffuse brain damage, and therefore with the generality of cognitive outcome, they do not take account of the effects of localized damage, or the fact that slight damage to some structures may have far more profound effects on function than more severe damage to others. For example, severe brain-stem injury leads to very long coma duration, yet may occur in injuries which cause little transfer of kinetic energy, and thus little diffuse damage (whether from direct contusion or from secondary compression as a result of intracranial haematoma). On the other hand, an injury which involves relatively slow crushing may cause severe persistent dysphasia but only brief coma and PTA. There are thus many exceptions to the correlational rule (in both directions), and rehabilitation needs to concern itself with all aspects of dysfunction. Several workers have already employed a different sort of classification (Annegers et al., 1980; Wang et al., 1986) in which contusion, haematoma and skull fracture are taken into account in the definitions of 'severe', 'moderate' and 'mild', in addition to Russell's criteria. Perhaps the importance of coma and PTA durations should be to indicate the probability of persisting cognitive dysfunction where this might otherwise pass unnoticed. But a more operational sort of classification may serve better in the planning of rehabilitation services. Thus the major groups of patients to be catered for are probably the following.

Group 1 The mildly or moderately injured who make a rapid and complete (or nearly complete) physical recovery. These patients need some weeks or even months (and often some advice or treatment) to recover from post-concussional symptoms (headache, dizziness, and noise intolerance), fatiguability, disturbances of behaviour (irritability, temper outbursts, phobic anxiety, lack of drive (particularly sexual), and subtle cognitive dysfunction (attention deficits and minor dysmnesias).

The main need for these individuals will be careful follow-up, so that appropriate advice can be given and treatment for any amenable dysfunctions can be arranged. Advice about return to work is particularly important, since they are especially vulnerable to losing their jobs if they return before adequate stamina has been regained.

Group 2 Those with injuries of any degree of severity who have significant physical or communication disorders which are slow to resolve. These patients may have any degree of cognitive dysfunction, and in addition they are likely to have the same spectrum of minor disorders as Group 1. It is important not to let these be overshadowed in planning treatment. However, this group will need quite lengthy physical and cognitive rehabilitation, with careful monitoring. They form one of the groups who will need an intensive and comprehensive head injury rehabilitation unit.

Group 3 Those with very long coma and very severe physical deficits. The majority of this group have severe brain-stem disorders, either from direct initial trauma, or from brain-stem distortion in the wake of raised intracranial pressure (from intracranial haemorrhage or brain swelling) – one subset of the so-called **second injury**. It is almost a corollary that many of them have not, in fact, suffered severe head injury, in the sense of diffuse concussive damage, and are cognitively well preserved, although this is often hidden by anarthria or the general appearance imposed by very severe physical disability.

They form the second group who need the full facilities of a rehabilitation unit. But they have two specific features which need to be taken into account. First, they are often able to go on gaining from intensive rehabilitation for a very long time (often 2 years or more). Second, there is some evidence to suggest they may have a **latent period**: such patients have been seen to respond very well to rehabilitation efforts 1 or 2 years after injury, or even later, when they have seemed to fail to respond to intensive therapy earlier. It may be that this group will do best with preventive rather than intensive rehabilitation in the first instance.

Group 4 Those with severe physical disorders who also have disorders of behaviour sufficient to make them unmanageable or unresponsive in standard rehabilitation settings. These patients clearly need the full range of rehabilitation treatments, but they also need treatment for the behavioural disorders. This cannot be achieved through sedation, both because this provides only temporary relief, and because sedation is incompatible with the business of active rehabilitation. These individuals therefore require a separate rehabilitation unit designed to cope with and treat behaviour disorders (including deficits of drive and motivation).

Group 5 Those with injuries of any severity who make reasonably good and rapid recoveries physically, but who have severe changes in behaviour, which make them unacceptable in standard social or treatment settings. They certainly require active treatment of the behaviour disorders, but invariably also need rehabilitation directed towards cognitive functioning, social and occupational skills and life management. Since the number of such patients is quite small, they can, with advantage, be treated together with Group 4, who share many of the same needs.

Group 6 Those who have suffered one or other of the very diffuse brain insults – hypoxia, ischaemia, hypoglycaemia or, in some cases, encephalitis with brain swelling. This is a most difficult group, for whom no solution appears to be currently available. The core members of the group are not head-injured, but head injury victims may also suffer a superimposed second injury of hypoxia (from throttling with a crash-helmet strap, or respiratory arrest) or ischaemic hypoxia (from shock or cardiac arrest, or from brain swelling or other severe rise in intracranial pressure). The result is often far more disastrous than a much more severe primary injury, because there results a strange state, combined with the more obvious effects of brain damage, which resembles nothing so much as the very gross hysterical states described by Charcot and his colleagues in the last century, and which usually involves indifference to reinforcement – indeed, to pleasure or pain.

Such patients cannot be managed effectively with the methods of behaviour modification (which often make them worse rather than better) to which Groups 4 and 5 have been shown to respond very well. In the present state of knowledge, they are a group who can be managed only with considerable frustration and difficulty, and they need the skills of nurses most versed in coping with the impossible. In other words, distasteful though it may seem, they need long-term psychiatric care. However, they present an enormous challenge, and it is to be hoped that intensive study of the problem may lead to some real solutions, as well as some new insights into brain function.

Group 7 Victims of head injury whose brain injury is so severe that they never recover what may properly be called consciousness – those suffering from what Jennett and Plum (1972) called **persistent vegetative state** (PVS). These patients require 'coma care' which may need to be very prolonged. They are few in number, and are to be found scattered around, usually not more than one in any hospital. In the last decade,

special coma care centres have grown up in the USA. The main opposition to such centres in the UK has been based on the belief that the carers for such patients would be under severe stress, and would be difficult to recruit. The main counter-argument has been that expertise is based upon experience. It is a particularly difficult question to resolve. Recently, however, there is evidence from the USA which strongly suggests that the families of these patients derive considerable benefit from such special units, principally because they no longer feel themselves pariahs, all patients in the unit being in the same predicament. This is a very powerful argument, although the small numbers involved pose confounding geographical problems in the UK. A further point which is gaining force as such units gather experience (although the phenomenon has long been enshrined in the literature) is that a few such patients can emerge from coma even after several years, and may even go on to make startling recoveries.

Social psychology of rehabilitation

Attitudes are deeply embedded in the individual, usually operate at an unconscious level and are likely to govern behaviour (especially non-verbal aspects), even in the presence of opposite conscious intentions (Sherif and Sherif, 1969; Reich and Adcock, 1976; Shakespeare, 1975, for reviews). They can be changed, but this is usually a slow process requiring consistent conditions. It is extremely difficult for a person to operate using more than one set of related attitudes at the same time, and in such conditions it is inevitably those deepest-rooted which most determine behaviour.

Attitudes have considerable impact on the process of rehabilitation. They need to be recognized, and taken into account when attempting to design a model service. Some of the ways in which attitudes affect the different groups of individuals involved in the process of rehabilitation are discussed below.

The head injury

Rehabilitation involves moving away from illness and disability towards independence and social well-being. If rehabilitation is to succeed fully, this idea has to be shared by the patient. This statement already highlights the problem: the very use of the word 'patient' tends to work against rehabilitation, in the mind of the sufferer as much as in the mind of the treater.

From our very early years, we learn that, when we are ill, we do not have to go to school (and therefore do not apply effort directed towards learning) and we are looked after without any expectation that things will be demanded of us. As a result, simply being in hospital, or being surrounded by the trappings of hospital and of medicine in general, is a powerful cue to passivity, and even to an ostensibly legitimate helplessness. Thus, in order to foster productive attitudes of mind in rehabilitation, we need to ensure that rehabilitation facilities symbolize, in their structure and decoration, the process of onward movement, away from illness and hospital, and towards the real world.

We must also ensure that the social environment carries the same message. It is important to avoid the possibility that those in rehabilitation compare themselves and their progress unfavourably with their fellows. This means paying attention to average rates of progress, which starkly distinguish, for example, those who have suffered severe head injury from those recovering from orthopaedic injuries.

Families

For the most part, the relatives of victims of head injury have pre-existing relationships with them which presuppose certain expectations about their behaviours, and long-confirmed patterns of respective emotional, social and practical roles. After injury, many of these expectations and patterns are no longer fulfilled – at least in the earlier stages of recovery. This leads to a whole set of mismatches which have to be resolved somehow. A wide variety of solutions is met with, and there are also many complex emotional and social disturbances which arise from failure to achieve a solution. In many instances, the form of the solution may lead to severe emotional strains, and to the breakdown of the relationship or to a distortion of it which inherently impedes rehabilitation.

In the case of spouses, for example, the stresses most frequently mentioned are the qualitative changes in the victim (He's not the man I married; It's distressing to wake up beside a stranger), and the inescapable need to take on additional roles which the injured person used to discharge automatically. The most usual outcomes of this situation are breakdown of the marriage (inevitably with much guilt, and often with open recrimination from the parental family), overt psychiatric illness in the spouse, or a radical change in the nature of the relationship, such that the injured person is accorded the role of a new and dependent child in the family.

In the case of unmarried victims (or, indeed, those whose marriages break down as a result of the effects of injury), the stresses fall usually upon the parental family. Here, the expectations are altogether different. Caring is, for most, an undeniable parental responsibility. But parents (especially mothers) usually find it a difficult enough task to 'let go' of their offspring in the first place, and being presented anew with a dependent son or daughter can lead to an unconscious desire to perpetuate the dependence, which can interfere with the more conscious wish to see the victim recover. This may even lead to covert sabotage of rehabilitation efforts.

For children, the stresses are different again, often involving either an almost 'play' reversal of roles, or an attempt to accept the injured parent as a peer – either of which can provoke resentful and angry responses from the injured parent once he or she begins to perceive it.

Such changes in relationships can not always be avoided, but the processes need to be understood if they and the suffering they engender are to be mitigated.

Staff

A central need for effective rehabilitation is that staff recognize and *believe in* the increases in functional competence that even the most severely head-injured can look forward to. Only then will they be comfortable in expecting them to make efforts at tasks currently beyond them, and to begin to take responsibility for themselves. Most members of the caring professions are specifically and extensively trained to *care for* people: when they work with individuals for whom the expectation is one of irreversible disability, they will care for them – and this is a concept which certainly does not include expecting them to take responsibility for themselves. To present staff trained in this way with a mixture of patients with radically different expected outcomes is to demand of them an impossible splitting of attitudes. In such circumstances it is inevitably the caring attitude which will prevail, and this can only be bad for those who have the potential for independence.

At a rather more subtle level, rehabilitation is prone to being undermined by attitudes implicit in the very professionalism of staff. Most of the professions involved are, by nature, based in hospitals, and many of their basic procedures have a hospital flavour. Probably the most obvious way in which a very clear separation between patients and staff is stated is the wearing of uniforms and badges. But there are many less explicit barriers, too. As with any profession, staff members unconsciously derive some of their security and confidence from various jargons, rituals and routines, yet to outsiders (and this includes the patients, their families and friends) these are quite alien and exclusive, often perplexing, and are no part of the real world to which we wish them to aspire.

Interpreting progress

When a person recovering from a severe head injury makes some distinct step in progress, there is often an unfortunate tendency for relatives (and sometimes rehabilitation staff, too) to focus upon it as though it were a goal rather than a step, and to encourage it with great enthusiasm. If the tempo of recovery is rapid, this may have no ill-effect, since further reacquisitions will soon replace it in their enthusiasms. But sometimes such reinforcement leads to the proud repetition of a maladaptive skill (a trick movement, for example), or to such concentration on the skill that its functional purpose is forgotten. Paul Jamie of the Nottingham rehabilitation services quoted a helpful example of this: his patient had spent so much time practising his skill at climbing stairs that, much later in recovery, he always knew how many stairs he had climbed, but rarely recalled why it was that he had gone upstairs.

The functional skills which we strive to reinstate in rehabilitation are, in the real world, merely means to the end of living, and are simply taken for granted by those without disabilities. This is well expressed in the dictum 'The most pervasive effect of a head injury is that the victim discovers that he has a head.' In rehabilitation, there is a continuing need to be resetting the sights 'up a notch'. Continual evaluation by all involved is vital, if counterproductive attitudes are to be replaced with productive ones.

3.2 QUESTIONS OF CONTENT

The range of areas of disturbed function presented by the head-injured demands an equal range of rehabilitative skills and methods. In some places, recognition of the range needed and of the primacy of psychological and psychosocial deficits has led to the relegation of physicians to the peripheral and almost trivial role of dealing with minor and intercurrent medical conditions. This shift has been aided by a lack of physicians with sufficient interest and expertise in the full breadth of the problems of head injury. However, knowledge and understanding of the mechanics and pathophysiology of injury, the nature of brain functions and of the 'person functions' they subserve, and the effects and treatment of neuropsychiatric disorders, are all essential ingredients in the processes of assessment and rehabilitation of the head-injured, and an appropriate physician is as necessary a member of the rehabilitation team as any.

Of course there is a need for physical therapies and treatments aimed at the correction of disorders of movement and speech, and these may need to continue for a short time, or for many months or even years. There is all too little information about which current treatments produce the best results, and there are reasons for thinking that the best methods are yet to be devised. Thus a major commitment of any service must be to the elaboration and evaluation of new approaches. It is also important to develop fitness and stamina.

Language disorders, both dysphasic and of higher level, need the skills of speech therapists and of neuropsychologists. Disorders of non-verbal aspects of language also need attention, and are best considered along with other elements of social skills training which can be pursued by interdisciplinary groups including speech therapists, occupational therapists, psychologists, social workers and nurses. With the head-injured, there is room in this spectrum for work on even more basic skills like rhythm, facial gesture, posture, and control of the range of vocal loudness.

Activities of daily living extend from personal care skills, through domestic and community skills, to the interpersonal aspects of work and recreation, and all need to be dealt with in rehabilitation. Of equal and complementary importance are those skills which incorporate both occupation and leisure activities.

Some techniques exist for the remediation of perceptual deficits, and methods of cognitive training are increasing, but both of these areas are in need of imaginative development. This is another field for cooperative efforts by occupational therapists and neuropsychologists, and there is likely to be much to be gained from collaboration in this with experimental and industrial psychologists, teachers in special education, graphic designers and computer scientists.

Behaviour disorders need treatment through behavioural techniques, and the (as yet) relatively unexplored anxiety disorders affecting the head-injured should be approached with behaviour and other psychological therapies.

It is now abundantly clear that family problems, both pre-existing and consequential, are of very great importance to outcome, and the expertise of social workers and social psychologists, as well as that of family members themselves, is likely to help lead to advances in their management.

3.3 QUESTIONS OF STRUCTURE

The case for *categorical* services

In trying to find ways of avoiding the deleterious effects of attitudes, we need to keep in mind clear distinctions between conditions which differ in a number of dimensions. Each of the features below evokes quite different (indeed opposing) attitudes to treatment.

1. The nature of the condition: congenital or life-long vs. later acquired;
2. The course of the condition: progressive vs. static vs. recovering;
3. The site of disease: non-cerebral vs. cerebral;
4. The rate of change: rapid vs. slow;
5. The pattern of brain damage: localized vs. diffuse (with or without localized);
6. The service offered: care vs. rehabilitation.

To harness the beneficial aspects of attitudes, it is essential to avoid trying to deal with mixed groups, at least in initial rehabilitation.

The disabilities of others serve as a mirror, and as a standard for one's own expectations. Of course the object of rehabilitation is to achieve reintegration in the real world, and the real world is full of mixtures. But the time for this is when the individual has acquired some belief in an improved future for himself. Moreover, it is necessary to remember that 'normal' individuals come across very few disabled people in the course of their everyday lives.

There is no doubt that it is possible for rehabilitation teams to cope with a very wide range of types of disability. However, it is not possible in those circumstances to develop the fullest understanding, or real expertise, of the particular problems presented by patients who fall into these categories. Nor is it possible to disentangle the different attitudes appropriate to the various groups. To achieve the best available outcome for the head-injured means providing the best rehabilitation, and that can be done only with special expertise, and with appropriate attitudes.

As was argued at the beginning of this chapter, if the present barrenness of rehabilitation services for the head-injured offers the opportunity for a new beginning, then we must be trying to establish the best ways of structuring our efforts, not just the possible. Clearly the best results are going to come from the practice of rehabilitating the head-injured as a special and separate group.

Stages of recovery and rehabilitation

It is useful to consider four periods following head injury, namely acute, intermediate, resettlement and long-term. These periods should be thought of as overlapping, rather than contiguous. Moreover, whether they are all applicable to any particular individual depends to a large extent on the severity of injury.

Acute

The acute period probably needs to be considered as extending from the time of injury to the end of the post-traumatic confusional period – what in retrospect we shall call PTA. This may be short, and coincide with the period of medical instability, or it may (in the case of more severe injuries) be very long, and much outlive that. The more prolonged it is, the more likely it becomes that the patient will present severe (though basically transient) behaviour management difficulties driven by the confusion itself.

It is clear that, as in so many cases, expertise through regular experience will lead to the most efficient decision-making, and to the best quality of care: when procedures become part of an established and frequently rehearsed routine, they are least likely to be overlooked. The corollary is that the best head injury service is likely to be one in which all patients presenting with head injury are under the management of one team, and admissions are concentrated in one place (i.e. one ward). The benefits of this sort of arrangement have been shown by a published study from Edinburgh (Miller and Jones, 1985), and also an (as yet) unpublished one from the Bristol Royal Infirmary. The benefits include a very substantial reduction in the number of admissions through safe and confident triage in the casualty departments; this represents a great saving in resources. Perhaps even more importantly, given recent evidence on the outcome after mild injuries not leading to admission to hospital (Rimel et al., 1981) such a structure allows referral for follow-up to be accomplished smoothly, thus both benefitting the victims, and also making it possible to extend outcome research to the whole population of the head-injured.

The concentration of patients in one area makes early rehabilitation consultations and assessments both easier (and therefore more likely actually to happen) and more efficient. The quality of communication between rehabilitation and ward staff is the greater because of the regular opportunities to learn each others' 'languages' and practices. It also allows the establishment of definite policies for dealing with the problems of dangerously disturbed behaviour.

Intermediate

Following admission to hospital because of head injury, it is virtually never reasonable for a person to return immediately to ordinary life and work. Indeed, for the majority there are considerable risks in doing so. Each case must be properly assessed first, to identify any problems needing treatment or **management through advice**. In relatively mild cases, this may be done by a standarized pre-discharge screening procedure (of the checklist variety), but if there are any question-marks at all, then at least one follow-up assessment is necessary.

Many patients will need to be followed-up for some months, some for years. If this is to be done effectively and efficiently, it needs to be done by a practised team – ideally the head injury follow-up clinic team. The essential team members are a doctor with a special interest in head injury rehabilitation (ideally a neuropsychiatrist), a psychologist (with a particular interest, and experience, in the neuropsychology of head injury) and a social worker (who should be a definite member of the team on a consistent basis). If the surgeon responsible for acute care were also involved, this would have the added benefit of eliminating parallel follow-up. Such a team creates the necessary focal point of the head injury service.

The clinic answers the needs of the majority of those suffering head injury. However, there are those who emerge from post-traumatic confusion (PTC), but still have significant deficits in a number of areas. They will be best served by a specialist rehabilitation centre. The patients thus receive the best possible management, staff gain solid expertise, research is greatly enhanced, and liaison with resettlement and care agencies is optimized. Those with severe behaviour disorders need a separate unit with a basically similar organization, but with special skill in behaviour management as well (Eames and Wood, 1985a; 1985b).

Recent extensive studies, both in the UK and abroad, make it clear that the largest single rehabilitation need after head injury is for cognitive retraining, and methods must be developed and refined. Many more patients are likely to need and benefit from such treatments than need the full panoply of rehabilitation, and it is probable that the most suitable service would therefore be one which functions autonomously, though in close liaison with the main unit.

Resettlement

Preparation and retraining for personal, domestic and occupational independence would be inherent in the operations of the main elements (general and behavioural head injury rehabilitation units, and follow-up clinic). For some victims such aims will never be fully achieved, and these will need long-term support or care of some degree. For others, however, various 'next step' facilities are needed to achieve the transition from intensive rehabilitation to independence, and these need to provide training in personal, occupational and recreational skills.

Long-term

For a small number of head injury victims (and the more organized and efficient the rehabilitation efforts, the smaller this number will be), various forms of long-term care and support will be needed.

At the top end of the spectrum, some will need supported accommodation, such as explicitly sympathetic lodgings, warden-supervised flats and group homes. A few will need more than this, because of irremediable physical disability. Some individuals, whilst not able to engage in remunerative work in the open market, will nevertheless be able to engage in sheltered work. It is necessary to ensure that not every workshop is organized as a rehabilitation facility, with a restricted length of stay: sheltered work often needs to continue until the person's retirement.

Patients in permanent PVS will need full, specialized medical and nursing care, some of them for several years. It must also be recognized that some persons with severe head injuries go on improving for many years, and thus some may ultimately reach a threshold at which a greater degree of independence becomes possible. It is therefore necessary to keep alive a set of attitudes open to such possibilities, and try to ensure that, in any long-term care setting, doors to the outside world can be readily opened.

It is apparent that, throughout the phases of recovery, all of the head-injured are likely to benefit from continued support of a most general kind – simply the knowledge that one is not forgotten can provide a moral boost.

3.4 CONCLUSIONS

It is apparent that the first need is for a coherent organization which takes account of the whole range of injuries, and seeks to identify and follow all victims until they have re-established themselves in as satisfactory a social niche as possible.

Management and treatment of persisting deficits will best be carried out in a dedicated (categorical) head injury unit, by an experienced and consistent team whose commitment is to this group. The team will have close links with both the acute treatment teams and the community services involved in resettlement and long-term care.

Such a unit will create a physical and cultural environment which is as close to the real world as possible, and which as far as possible hides those features of medical care which it is necessary to incorporate. This is the real answer to the arguments about institutional versus community rehabilitation: only a dedicated unit can provide proper interdisciplinary rehabilitation, accumulate expertise, undertake research, and answer the needs of cost-effectiveness; it avoids being institutional by being modelled on the real world in its outward appearances, and need be no less a part of the community than, say, a residential training college.

One of its essential features must be interdisciplinary team working: staff must expect to allow a degree of blurring and sharing of roles, and to learn and develop new skills which may be outside their normal professional requirements and experience. They will recognize that all disciplines have a part to play in the process, and none is any more essential than any other. They will also appreciate that there remains much to be learned, and that insights and advances may require contributions from fields not traditionally associated with rehabilitation.

REFERENCES

Annegers, J.F., Grabow, J.D., Groover, R.V. et al. (1980) Seizures after head trauma: a population study. Neurology, 30: 683–89.

Berrol, S., Rappaport, M., Cope, D.N. et al. (1982) Severe Head Trauma: a Comprehensive Medical Approach, Institute for Medical Research, Santa Clara Valley Medical Centre (751 South Bascom Avenue, San Jose, California 95128).

Brooks, N. (1984) Closed Head Injury, Oxford University Press.

Brooks, N., Campsie, L., Symington, C. et al. (1986) A five year outcome of severe blunt head injury: a relatives view. J. Neurol., Neurosurg. and Psychiat., 49: 764–70.

Bryden, J. (1985) Epidemiology of head injury, Paper presented to Medical Disability Society, Nottingham, July 1985.

Eames, P. and Wood, R.L. (1985a) Rehabilitation after severe brain injury: a special-unit approach to behaviour disorders. Int. Rehabil. Med., 7: 130–33.

Eames, P. and Wood, R.L. (1985b) Rehabilitation after severe brain injury: a follow-up study of a behaviour modification approach. J. Neurol., Neurosurg. Psychiat., 48: 613–19.

Jennett, B. and Plum, F. (1972) Persistent vegetative state after brain damage. Lancet, i, 734–37.

London, P.S. (1967) Some observations on the course of events after severe injury of the head. *Ann. R. Coll. Surg. Eng.*, **41**, 460–79.

Miller, J.D. and Jones, P.A. (1985) The work of a Regional Head Injury Service. *Lancet*, **i**, 1141–44.

Reich, B and Adcock, C. (1976) *Values, Attitudes and Behaviour Change*, Methuen, London.

Rimel, R.W., Giordani, B, Barth, J.T. *et al.* (1981) Disability caused by minor head injury. *Neurosurgery*, **9** (3), 221–28.

Royal College of Physicians (1986) Physical handicap in 1986 and beyond. *J. Roy. Coll. Phys.*, **20**, 3, 161–93.

Russell, W.R. and Smith, A. (1961) Post-traumatic amnesia in closed head injury. *Arch. Neurol.*, **5**, 16–29.

Shakespeare, R. (1975) *The Psychology of Handicap*, Methuen, London.

Sherif, M. and Sherif, C.W. (1969) *Social Psychology*, Harper & Row, New York.

Teasdale, G. and Jennett, B. (1974) Assessment of coma and impaired consciousness. A practical scale. *Lancet*, **ii**, 81–84.

Teasdale, G. and Mendelow, D. (1984) Pathophysiology of head injuries. In *Closed Head Injury: Psychological, Social and Family Consequences* (N. Brooks, ed.), Oxford University Press.

Wang, C.-C., Schoenberg, B.S., Li, S.-C. *et al.* (1986) Brain injury due to trauma: epidemiology in urban areas of the People's Republic of China. *Arch. Neurol.*, **43**: 570–72.

Wood, R.L. and Eames, P. (1981) Application of behaviour modification in the treatment of traumatically brain-injured adults. In *Applications of Conditioning Theory* (G. Davey, ed.), Methuen, London.

4

Head injury rehabilitation: towards a 'model' service

Peter Eames

A coherent, comprehensive rehabilitation service for spinal injury in the UK now exists more or less nationwide. The small number of victims involved, and the appropriately small number of units, impose problems of distance, both for families and for the business of communication between centres and referrers, but these are inevitable, and are more or less accepted for that reason.

Despite significant head injuries outnumbering spinal injuries by something of the order of 40 to 1, there is virtually no coherent rehabilitation service for them anywhere in the country. Worldwide, great strides in the understanding of the problems of head injury are being made, and there is a rapidly increasing awareness that 'something needs to be done'. The growing pressure from both professionals and the victims of head injury and their families are inevitably going to lead to service developments. There is therefore a pressing need for creative thinking and design, so that these developments do not simply reproduce the deficiencies of past approaches.

There have never been many rehabilitation centres in the UK, and only a very few have developed particular interest, experience and expertise in the problems of brain injury. In the last year or two, the two leading centres have shrunk, and are no longer able to treat patients from outside their catchment populations. One of these centres, the Joint Services Medical Rehabilitation Unit, recently moved from Chessington to Headley Court, illustrates the problem: in the last few years, particularly because of consequences of the Falklands campaign, they have had to refuse admission to civilian patients, turning down some fifty requests a year.

At the same time, over the last decade there has been increasing evidence (mostly from abroad, but also from this country) that intensive and prolonged rehabilitation can dramatically improve the long-term outcome. Designed to improve the whole range of deficits of the head-injured, rehabilitation can be successful even for the most severely injured, in terms of the degree of independent living achieved, and thus of the quantity of support services needed (Najenson et al., 1974; Berrol et al., 1982; Eames and Wood, 1985; Jacobs, 1985.)

The distribution of the population of the UK is far from homogeneous, and it seems unlikely that any one blueprint for a comprehensive head injury service could perfectly answer the needs of every area. However, it does seem likely that an underlying standard pattern of management would be appropriate. This chapter offers an example of a model service, based on the principles discussed in the previous chapter. It must be stressed that the model is based on British needs and existing health care delivery institutions; although it may therefore have little direct relevance for other countries, the exercise in general may provoke helpful ideas.

4.1 SCOPE AND ELEMENTS OF THE MODEL

Objectives of the service

It is necessary to distinguish four main objectives.

1. To protect and enhance the quality of life, and emotional and social wellbeing, of the injured person and of the family;
2. To increase the expertise of the treaters, and thus the quality and effectiveness of treatment and the level of work satisfaction;
3. To study the effectiveness of the service, and of treatment methods used and developed (in other words, research);
4. To increase efficiency, especially in terms of the long-term cost-effectiveness of treatment, taking due account of the costs of permanent care, and of long-term impacts on the economic viability of the injured.

An important aspect of trying to achieve these aims, and one which is most lacking at present, is the need to cater for as large a proportion of head injury victims as possible. Very many patients with potentially avoidable or remediable problems fall through the net. A strategy of considerable power to prevent this is to ensure that there are as few pieces of string as possible! In practice this means creating a system and an accepted and recognized pattern of flow for patients suffering head injury, which involve only a limited and specified group of clinicians.

Principles of structuring the model

1. Establishing a funnel. In every district hospital accepting accident cases, the acute management of head injuries should become the responsibility of one team, so that decision-making can be simplified, training of juniors enhanced, and identification for the purpose of follow-up ensured.

2. Coping with dangerous behaviour. In the acute phase, there is a need to establish clear, planned ways of dealing with the problems of dangerously disturbed behaviour. This is not a frequent problem, but it generates a great deal of alarm and, indeed, bad feeling when it does appear. If the patient is still in need of active medical or surgical treatment, then it is the acute hospital which is needed, and there is no alternative to sedation. However, this must be sufficient to produce a controlled, stuporose, or at least fully compliant patient, and must avoid, wherever possible, drugs known to retard and prevent neuronal recovery, or to increase the likelihood of epilepsy: what is needed, then, is a careful and collaborative agreed standard procedure.

A much greater problem is the patient who is medically stable, but who is still confused, especially if physical disabilities are slight. If there is behavioural disorder, it nearly always poses threats to the safety of other patients and of staff. Such patients can be effectively nursed only by those with special skills in managing difficult behaviour, and this means psychiatric nurses. Whilst it can be argued that such problems are not psychiatric, it is inescapably true that psychiatrists are in control of the people with the necessary skills for dealing with it. Again the need is for an agreed procedure, guaranteeing the speedy removal of such a patient to wherever is deemed (as a general feature of the procedure, not in each individual case) the most appropriate setting. Effectively, because of the organization of responsibility for psychiatric in-patient services, this means the agreement and participation of a specific consultant psychiatrist with facilities at his or her disposal for the admission of acutely disturbed patients. Given the small numbers to be expected, the policy should not be constrained by the question of catchment areas. Undoubtedly such a plan would generate much goodwill.

3. Establishing a follow-up clinic. To provide the focal point, a distinct head injury follow-up clinic should be established, manned by a permanent team (head injury physician, social worker and neuro-psychologist) working in collaboration with the acute team, and also with the head injury therapists in the acute hospital. (Clinic is meant in the functional rather than the architectural sense.)

4. *Separation of the head-injured from other patients.* Formal rehabilitation units for the head-injured should be developed separately from those patients with other sorts of disorders, and should be located, as far as possible, away from hospitals. If no alternative can be found to siting them within hospital campuses, they should nevertheless be designed to be as non-institutional, and as separate from hospital routines, as bureaucracy can be persuaded to allow.

5. *Staffing.* Such statistics as are available suggest that two or three units suitably placed geographically, each with 20 beds and the potential for the same number of day patients, would cover the needs of a region. In planning such a unit, it would be vital to recognize that many patients would need lengthy rehabilitation, and that there could be no standard duration of treatment. Nursing such a unit would require probably only four nurses per shift (two trained and, say, one assistant and one student nurse). There would be considerable advantage in planning for joint staffing, with a mixture of general and psychiatric trained nurses. There are good reasons for thinking that at least a proportion of behavioural disorders are unwittingly fostered by inappropriate reinforcement through unfamiliarity with techniques of management, and it is likely that the incidence of persisting disorders could be reduced by the incorporation of nurses experienced in such techniques. Moreover, both established and trainee general nurses would benefit by practical learning of the skills, and psychiatric nurses by achieving confidence with physical and communication disorders.

Among therapy staff, the patient numbers quoted would need four or five physiotherapists, two speech therapists, and probably five occupational therapists (one of whom should be experienced particularly in work aspects, and two of whom should have psychiatric experience to facilitate work with social skills, social anxiety problems and perceptual and cognitive training). The addition of an educational therapist would harness the advantages recently demonstrated in Nottingham, and elsewhere. The extensive need for cognitive retraining should be met by the addition of a psychology technician working under the direction of the neuropsychologists.

The other needs of the rehabilitation team would best be met if the follow-up clinic teams took the medical, psychological and social work responsibilities for the unit, assisted by whatever trainees were currently attached to the clinics. This would also ensure ready communication between the various elements of the service.

All staffing should be as stable as can be achieved. If the policy is to rotate staff for purposes of clinical experience then sufficient time in each location should be allowed for this experience to be worthwhile.

6. *Special behavioural units.* A special unit for those with severe behaviour disorders persisting beyond the acute phase would need a basically similar organization. However, the need for psychiatric nurses would be greater, the best establishment being charge nurses with double qualification, assisted by psychiatric nurses. This unit would need more psychologist time than the main unit, and this would be best met by having a junior clinical psychologist committed half-time, under the direction of the clinic neuropsychologists. The demands of disordered behaviour and of behavioural treatment would require the same number of nurses as for the main rehabilitation unit, although the maximum number of patients should not exceed about 15. However, numbers of therapy staff would be substantially lower: two physiotherapists, one speech therapist, two occupational therapists and an education therapist would be appropriate.

Such limited evidence as is available suggests that probably only about nine patients needing such a unit would appear in a region each year. Since treatment time is likely to be about 1 year on average, it is clear that a special behavioural unit for the head-injured would be under-used by one region alone. The options for the solution of the problems posed by these patients would seem to be either to adopt a policy of buying-in to some other organization providing such a facility (which is very likely to be in the private sector, where the only two such units currently exist), or to establish units to cover the needs of two neighbouring regions, sooner or later seeking DHSS support for them.

7. *Team work.* In all of these elements, the emphasis should be on interdisciplinary team working: staff must expect to allow a degree of blurring and sharing of roles, and to learn and develop new skills which may be outside their normal professional requirements and experience.

8. *Using resources.* In the interest of efficiency and cost-effectiveness, it should be recognized that a great deal of professional time and effort is already being spent on many of these patients. This effort is often ineffective, partly because individual staff deal with only a few such

patients, and thus do not develop expertise, and partly because conditions rarely allow sufficiently lengthy rehabilitation for major or lasting achievements. The corollary is that, as long as all the districts involved were prepared to work together, many of the necessary elements of a comprehensive service could be achieved by redeploying staff and services already available, thus greatly reducing the need for extra funding. This aim can also be furthered by the exploration of new methods based on group treatment.

9. Preparation for community resettlement.   Many facilities needed for community resettlement already exist or are being developed. The Manpower Services Commission disposes not only of the assessment and retraining facilities of the Employment Rehabilitation Centres (ERCs), but also of the access to a wide variety of countrywide retraining courses. For some patients, there is advantage in exploring intermediate training opportunities in industrial therapy departments and centres. The increasing activities of the Shaw Trust are most helpful in supporting effectively sheltered employment.

There is a need also for what might be called accommodation training. To some extent this is available in some of the housing association projects. The National Head Injuries Association (Headway) is becoming actively involved in similar projects aimed specifically at the needs of the head-injured. The essential problem which needs to be recognized is that actual independence involves stresses which cannot be adequately simulated in the main rehabilitation settings; almost by definition, the individual has to be *really* on his or her own if viability is to be tested. It may be that specific testing accommodation will need to be developed, though it should be possible for this to be a part of a wider venture.

To exploit these various possibilities, the main requirement is for good, open communication and liaison initiated and sustained by the head injury units.

10. Long-term care.   The Cheshire Foundation and some of the independent Housing Associations are developing a specific interest in the long-term care of the head-injured. Headway has such an interest nationally. It may prove possible, at the local level, to exploit the fact that many victims come to dispose of funds awarded for their long-term care needs, which could perhaps be pooled for the purpose of setting up suitable life settings for themselves and, indeed, others. Community Service Volunteers can be an added source of help.

11. Special units for those unresponsive to treatment.   It is likely that a very few victims of brain injury (including some with head injury) will be able to be cared for (and indeed tolerated) only in long-term psychiatric settings, once lengthy rehabilitative efforts have proved to be in vain. The potential mutually deleterious interactions between such patients and other long-term psychiatric groups might be avoided by establishing a special unit for the former, which could well cater for some other problem groups (patients with presenile dementias, for example), but which would nevertheless allow close study of these special problems, and thus lead to more fruitful treatment approaches.

12. Coma care.   It seems clear that any specialist coma care unit would need to be established within a general hospital, associated closely with intensive care facilities, but also in regular contact with the head injury teams, so that appropriate steps could be taken if signs of recovery of consciousness appeared.

13. Social support.   There is a need for a very general kind of social support, for both the head-injured and their families, over the whole period of recovery and rehabilitation. This is a function which Headway seems ideally placed and constituted to fulfil, but clear involvement with that organization by the professionals of the head injury teams is undoubtedly an important and powerful sustaining force.

4.2 SUMMARY OF THE MODEL

1. The funnel.   All head-injured patients presenting at hospital are dealt with by a specific acute surgical team, thus ensuring identification of the whole population, adequate follow-up, efficient and cost-effective admission policies and guidelines, and valuable on-going research. Patients not admitted are referred to the head injury follow-up clinic within a week or two.

2. Acute care.   The surgical team is augmented by the follow-up clinic team, thus strengthening continuity, and allowing planning of subsequent rehabilitation from an early stage. Specific policies are established for the management of behavioural problems. Acute hospital therapists are identified as a specific team involved with head injury, and thus gain solid experience and expertise, liaising with the follow-up clinic team.

3. The follow-up clinic.   This team (head injury physician, social worker and neuropsychologist) follows up all head-injured patients, whether admitted or not, until they re-achieve independent social and occupational roles. Responsibility for on-going research is taken by the team.

4. *The head injury rehabilitation unit.* This unit serves a number of districts, whose clinic teams contribute to its management. It deals with both inpatients and day patients, and continues rehabilitation for as long as is necessary to achieve the best possible outcome.

5. *The behavioural unit.* This unit provides both treatment of behaviour disorders, and continuing rehabilitation. The same district clinic teams are involved as necessary.

6. *The cognitive retraining unit.* This unit offers cognitive training to the two units, and also to patients with home-based computer systems, through the telephone network. It collects and analyses data to monitor individuals' progress and needs, and for research in order to refine and develop methods.

7. *The coma care unit.* This unit accepts patients in extended coma or persistent vegetative state, aiming to provide continuing support for families, and to arrange referral for further rehabilitation of those who emerge from coma.

8. *Resettlement and long-term care.* The district teams develop and maintain close liaison with community services for work and accommodation, both statutory and independent, and ensure smooth transitions from active rehabilitation. Strong links are maintained with local Headway groups.

4.3 NEEDS FOR DETAILED PLANNING

The structural details of a head injury rehabilitation service must depend to some extent on research into the actual size of the problem in the given area and other local factors. Below is a list of steps required for ultimate planning. However, the problem is an urgent one, and provided initial solutions are developed as far as possible by means of redeploying facilities and staff already available, there is no justification for delaying until all information is available: the means of accurate planning, and the establishment of a workable provisional service, can and should be pursued concurrently.

Moreover, one of the advantages of a model is that its implementation can serve as a pilot study, at the same time as it is providing a service. There is much to be said, from a national point of view, for the idea of implementing the model in a few areas (perhaps with recognizably different geographical constraints), in order to test it out, and assess its strengths and weaknesses.

Research

1. Most urgently needed is an extensive and accurate study of the numbers of head injuries, the proportions of different severities, and the current disposals and outcomes. This whole question is bedevilled by the fact that the incidence of injury is not static (for example, substantial reductions have occurred following seat-belt legislation). Nevertheless, the most suitable approach would seem to be a study of, say, a one-year cohort of patients arriving at hospital with head injury. The year chosen should allow a follow-up period of long enough to give reasonable outcome data. Moreover, the study should involve an area large enough and of varied enough population to allow accurate extrapolations.
2. An enquiry should be made of all hospitals and long-stay homes in the region to establish how many patients are currently needing care for PVS and for severe physical deficits from head injury and other brain injuries. (If this was done widely at regional level, the pooled results of all the regions would, of course, give a very full national view.)
3. An enquiry should be made of all psychiatric, psychogeriatric and mental handicap hospitals to establish how many patients are currently being cared for with severe behavioural disorders conse-quent on head injury and on diffuse brain insults.
4. A directory of 'Who's Who' should be constructed of local person-nel currently offering services of any sort to victims of head injury. This should include at least health, social, educational, manpower and independent resources.

Service

1. Discussions should be opened between all consultant staff who admit acute head injury patients, to try to establish a system of funnelling all such patients into a restricted area, and under the care of as small a number of consultants (and therefore trainees) as possible.
2. Discussions should be stimulated through the local divisions of psychiatry to establish the best advice on adequate and undamag-ing sedation, and other strategies for the management of

behaviourally disturbed, acutely ill head injury patients, and also to establish an agreed permanent contingency plan for the temporary management of those patients who are no longer surgically ill, but whose cognitive disorder leads to disturbed behaviour which cannot be coped with in an acute surgical setting. The Royal College of Psychiatrists has a special interest group, liaison with which might best produce a nationally agreed set of guidelines.

3. Provisional district head injury rehabilitation teams should be established. The team's functions should include manning the head injury follow-up clinic (to which are referred all patients discharged after admission with head injury, and also those patients seen in the casualty department with a definite head injury, but not admitted), and liaising with the consultant(s) in charge of the acute head injury area in order to organize early, and plan for later, rehabilitation. Several district teams would be centrally involved in the planning and establishing of the (area) head injury rehabilitation units.

4. A survey should be made of all facilities in the area to generate ideas about possible locations of the categorical head injury rehabilitation unit. This should include careful consideration of facilities (or parts of facilities) which are due for closure: often there are parts of properties which might be very suitable, and which would be 'detachable' from the main property, and able to function as small, separate units. Such a process might call for a 'saving forgone' by the district health authority, but the effective cost would be very much smaller than that of establishing a unit *de novo*.

5. Local clinical psychologists should be encouraged to explore ways of setting up cognitive retraining programs.

6. A local conference should be convened, involving all medical specialists currently engaged in any way in head injury care or rehabilitation, and all community physicians to establish a plan for the structure and functioning of a comprehensive service. The principle of minimizing new costs through redeployment of existing resources will require considerable collaboration between districts, since numbers do not justify the idea of district rehabilitation units.

REFERENCES

Berrol, S., Rappaport, M., Cope, D.N. et al. (1982) *Severe Head Trauma: a Comprehensive Medical Approach*, Institute for Medical Research, Santa Clara Valley Medical Center (751 South Bascom Avenue, San Jose, California 95128).

Bryden, J. (1985) *Epidiomiology of head injury*, Paper presented to Medical Disability Society, Nottingham, July 1985.

Eames, P. and Wood, R.L. (1985) Rehabilitation after severe brain injury: a follow-up study of a behaviour modification approach. *J. Neurol. Neurosurg. Psychiat.*, **48**, 613–19.

Jacobs, H.E. (1985) *The family as a therapeutic agent: long term rehabilitation for traumatic head injury patients*, UCLA School of Medicine, Los Angeles.

Najenson, T., Mendelson, L., Schechter, I. *et al.* (1974) Rehabilitation after severe head injury. *Scand. J. Rehabil. Med.*, **6**, 5–14.

5   Rehabilitation in the community

Chris Evans and Betty Skidmore

There is no generally available facility for the rehabilitation of brain-damaged patients in the UK. There are isolated pockets of excellence and enthusiasm but wide areas of neglect. Ideally, there should be specialized centres established to deal with these patients, similar to those which care for paraplegics. No major handicap is easy to look after, even if it is solely a physical problem. However, looking after those who have sustained severe brain damage is harder because of the alteration of personality, usually for the worse. For most carers it is seen as a lifetime sentence. Even those who start the task with all the love and care possible may falter in looking after a seemingly ungrateful, and unfamiliar person. Most of the victims are young, with a normal life expectancy, making the future for the carers even more bleak. The problem is growing because seat belt and crash helmet laws have ensured more survivors of accidents, some with brain damage. This is not to devalue the fact that there are fewer deaths, but to point out that the consequences of such survival have not yet been fully appreciated.

These problems are at last receiving some attention, but since it is probable that the numbers of such survivors will increase swiftly it will not be possible to build and develop sufficient new inpatient units; other strategies will, therefore, have to be devised. This chapter attempts to define rehabilitation, describes present and proposed plans for management of head injuries in Cornwall (in the extreme south-west of England), lists existing facilities, and outlines the difficulties experienced in producing a coherent strategy. It then details a local response to the challenge, and gives reasons which suggest that the concept of community-based rehabilitation could give a better result than can be achieved in hospitals or conventional rehabilitation units.

The proposals depend in part on the establishment and use of community rehabilitation teams (CRTs). This is a new idea, with potential to allow earlier discharge from hospital and better resettlement in the community. Even though not all the sequelae of a head injury can be managed in the community, arguments will be offered to support the establishment of a community-based programme rather than to try developing only residential or outpatient-based schemes. It is essential to success that community-based services must be fully funded and staffed, and supported by hospitals, primary care teams and social services.

5.1 GENERAL CONSIDERATIONS

There is a trend, which is gathering momentum, towards care in and by the community. It has become more apparent over the last decade, is occurring faster abroad than in the UK, and is particularly apparent in the United States. It is partly due to a recoil from the medical model to an alternative one, aided by the realization that hospital care alienates people with handicaps from their families, social networks and their community structures. In addition, large centralized hospitals catering for districts with populations of about a quarter of a million cause major economic and transport problems for patients, their relatives and friends. This is most marked in rural areas such as Cornwall.

5.2 DEFINITION OF REHABILITATION

There has been a great deal of work and thought on defining rehabilitation during the last few years. In particular a working party and steering committee have been convened in Birmingham for the West Midlands Regional Health Authority with the remit to advise on the development of rehabilitation services. A quote from the report states:

> The Steering Committee, like the Working Party before it, gave careful thought to the meaning of the word 'rehabilitation'. There are three main components; medical, social and employment and education. They cannot be separated; they must be combined with continuity between them. None of the available definitions is entirely satisfactory; a description is preferable.
>
> Rehabilitation is a process intended to enable a disabled person to play as active, independent and satisfying a part in everyday life as possible. For some this means the medical and other care that enables them to resume all their previous activities after temporary disablement from illness or injury. For others, disablement continues although its level may fluctuate. The objective should be to try to prevent handicap from getting worse and to try, wherever possible,

to enhance both residual capabilities and the range of activities to choose from. Disabilities may date from birth or they may follow a period of normal development and functioning. Different methods of rehabilitation will be required, depending on the need to acquire fresh skills or to relearn or adapt old ones. Individuals should be encouraged to make their own decisions about their lives. The acquisition or restoration of independence must involve 'stretching and challenging disabled persons rather than over-protecting them' (London, 1987).

The rehabilitation process can be divided into three phases. The first is when most effort is directed towards altering the condition of the patient (or client). The second is directed towards changing the environment, and the third attempts to change attitudes. These attitudes may be of the handicapped persons themselves, but they are also concerned with those of society. All these aspects of rehabilitation are important in discussing brain damage, and it is argued that the community is the place where most of the work can be done. Again, while attempts have been made here to analyse different aspects of rehabilitation it must be stressed that in practice they will be closely integrated.

Rehabilitation should be taking place continually after a head injury, during each of the three stages of recovery. First is the acute stage, which takes place in hospital; second is post-acute rehabilitation, often in specialized ward, or inpatient rehabilitation unit where available; finally is long-term follow-up care, normally shared by outpatient departments and the community, but with no organized or active role for the latter.

It is helpful to put a scale to the programme. Table 5.1 analyses the patients referred to the rehabilitation consultant in Cornwall from September 1983 to December 1986. It will be seen that there are two main categories; those whose handicap has been present since birth, and those who have acquired handicap in later life. The largest group in this second category is of those who have survived CVA (stroke). Multiple sclerosis and chronic back pain are also frequently referred. Severe head injury is a major problem; it is about three times more frequently referred than paraplegia and tetraplegia combined. There are about 70 patients who have suffered major brain damage from head injury in Cornwall now. This is a minimum figure, since it is unlikely that all patients will be referred to the consultant in rehabilitation. It does, however, give an order of magnitude for the district (about 350 000) which accords with recent national and local estimates. (Bryden, in preparation; Wade and Langton Hewer, 1987).

Table 5.1. Patients referred to the rehabilitation consultant in Cornwall from September 1983 to December 1986

Diagnosis	Number
Cerebrovascular accident (CVA)	339
Multiple sclerosis	159
Head injury	**76**
Cerebral palsy	39
Paraplegia	27
Motor neurone disease	24
Brachial plexus	16
Parkinson's disease	14
Muscular dystrophy	12
Spina bifida	12
Subarachnoid haemorrhage	**11**
Huntington's chorea	10
Tetraplegia	9
TOTAL	748

On the other hand, the numbers of patients with the sequelae of head injury do not justify specialized head injury units in an area of this size, so it seems inevitable that mixed units are essential. The resources and knowledge of the CRTs are a major step because they permit earlier discharge into the community with the confidence that the original concepts of rehabilitation will be preserved.

For an effective rehabilitation service the following aspects need to be considered:

1. Support for the acute services in the district general hospital;
2. Residential rehabilitation facility with community outreach;
3. Workshops providing training, work assessment and experience;
4. Hostel accommodation with facilities for daily living and social skills;
5. Community-based teams to coordinate local programmes;
6. Resource centres supporting problems of residual handicap;
7. Multidisciplinary management services;
8. Research into, and evaluation of, services and individual programmes.

The intention should be to provide a residential rehabilitation service only until the individual can return to his own home and then to provide the person with a full community programme and support. At first sight this seems a statement of the obvious, but it is not common practice, the difficulty usually being the disintegration of the outpatient programme. If it were done properly it would enable progress after the acute and post-acute stages to be initiated and continued within the patient's original environment as soon as possible.

The rehabilitation service developing in Cornwall is a combination of residential and community-based rehabilitation teams. There is increasing emphasis being placed on the use of community facilities, and of extending the hospital services into the community. Overlap is avoided by the use of key workers, and the regular meeting of the CRTs.

5.3 MANAGEMENT PATTERNS

The management of the acute stage devolves into one of four specialities.

1. General surgery
2. Orthopaedic surgery
3. Accident and emergency surgery
4. Anaesthetics

Patients in Cornwall assessed as needing neurosurgery are transferred, when fit to travel, to the neurosurgical unit in Plymouth, and readmitted when surgery is complete and the medical condition stable. As in many other parts of the country the allocation of the individual patient will mainly depend upon any associated injuries, and whether resuscitation is needed.

Policies are now under discussion which it is hoped will, when finally agreed, include the following points:

Initial assessment

Head injuries will be categorized as severe if the duration of unconsciousness exceeds 6 hours. Such cases will be introduced to the rehabilitation service at this stage. Physiotherapists, occupational therapists, speech therapists, clinical psychologist and social worker should be involved with the patient and the family or other carers.

Long-term programmes

Where it is likely that there will be long-term effects the patient is transferred from intensive treatment unit or resuscitation unit direct to the Cornwall Stroke and Rehabilitation Unit (CSRU). Criteria for transfer are that medical stability must have been achieved, and arterial and venous lines successfully withdrawn. The CSRU will cope with nasogastric tubes, catheters, and stable tracheostomies.

Rehabilitation at this stage should be intensive; ideally there should be sufficient nursing and paramedical staff to permit a full programme of activities planned on a 9 a.m. to 5 p.m. daily basis even if not all patients can accept all the programme at the beginning. The system should not fall apart at weekends but may use relatives and friends wherever possible. If this scale of programme does not exist, then the group of patients who have major brain damage but are physically mobile will become bored and aggressive very rapidly, and often insist on premature self-discharge home where they cause much disruption for just the same reasons. This is usually to their subsequent detriment. It is essential to include comprehensive clinical psychological assessment and treatment at this early stage. It is important to keep and develop the support of the family, and to introduce help from the community at this stage as well.

Discharge

When inpatient intensive rehabilitation produces no further improvement (and this time is very variable) most patients go home. Discharge plans are discussed by members of the team with the relatives, and with any department which may have a part in subsequent rehabilitation. Given the patient's agreement they will also be presented to their local CRT.

Follow-up

Follow-up is arranged either in the CSRU, at a designated clinic or as part of ordinary outpatients at the peripheral hospital. The results of these clinics provide the medical input to the CRTs. It is hoped that the clinic at the CSRU will also be the screening centre for patients with severe head injury who are not considered sufficiently handicapped to need transfer to the CSRU directly, but who may be potentially handicapped.

5.4 EXISTING REHABILITATION UNITS

The rehabilitation service has three residential units which share in the management of head injury.

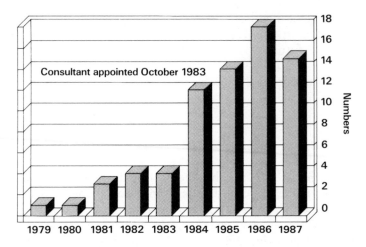

Figure 5.1 Severe head-injured patients: annual admissions to CSRU.

Cornwall Stroke and Rehabilitation Unit (CSRU) at City Hospital, Truro. This unit has 16 beds and virtually always has some patients there who are suffering the after-effects of head injury. Their numbers have increased sharply in the last 4 years, and about 18 patients with traumatic brain damage were admitted during 1986. This probably reflects a change of transfer policy rather than an increase in the number of head injuries who survive (Fig. 5.1).

Kerensa, a social services rehabilitation unit at St Austell. This unit is run by the social services and provides 24 residential and 24 non-residential places. There are extensive workshops offering a wide range of crafts and trades. Three bungalows in the grounds are used as half-way houses between residential care and return to the community. The unit provides a flexible pattern of care designed for the individual. It is intended to be informal and residents are encouraged to make as many decisions for themselves as possible. The unit also participates in many local community activities, and has strong links with technical college, employers, voluntary organizations and local sports facilities. Social skills, self-help are also encouraged and activities of daily living introduced where needed.

The Young Disabled Unit, Marie Therese House, Hayle. This has 12 beds and provides programmed care. It currently supports 70 families in the community, mostly with multiple sclerosis, but does look after two patients as long-stay residents who have suffered severe brain damage. One has been in a coma for 2 years. If trends in the US are repeated in the UK then coma care will be an increasing problem for the future.

All three units maintain links with the community, both directly, and through the CRTs.

5.5 PROBLEMS OF RESIDENTIAL UNITS

The medical model of care has been criticized in many quarters because it can create more problems than it solves, particularly when it has to help with problems of long-term rehabilitation after brain damage. It is in many ways antipathetic to aspirations for independence (Kennedy, 1980; Zola, 1977; Friedson, 1975; Illich, 1977). Hitherto pleas for change have largely gone unheard, and where heard, unheeded. However, Harrison (1986) in a comprehensive monograph on residential care for young people with physical handicaps (of whom head-injured patients form a significant number) not only outlines present deficiencies in residential care but does so with the authority of the Royal College of Physicians behind him. This can only confirm that in the UK the time is now ripe for these problems to be addressed.

Since Goffman published *Asylums* (1961) there has been an increasing awareness of the problems caused by segregating handicapped people from their community. He points out that most people have different areas to work, sleep, rest and play in. These areas are important, but tend to overlap and lose distinction in many institutions, even those designed to manage the after-effects of head injury. Furthermore the activities are monitored by staff who have authority to make all decisions for those in their care. Indeed, during the early stages of recovery after a head injury this has to be the case. For how long, and what degree of authority staff should assume are legitimate subjects for debate. It is surprisingly easy to delegate decision-making responsibilities to others in such circumstances, even for individuals who have not sustained brain damage. Given, however, that decision-making capabilities are essential for most people, and accepting that they will inevitably be compromised in the acute stage after head injury while the patient is unconscious or semiconscious, it seems unhelpful to perpetuate this state any longer than necessary. Furthermore, researchers have documented the effect known as 'learned helplessness' (Abramson *et al.* 1978). The individual learns that he is impotent to affect the environment. This leads to apathy, moroseness and the rejection of any attempt by others to change anything.

Lazarus and Monat (1977) also emphasize the need for people to perceive themselves to be in charge of their own actions, behaviour and future. They posit that when environmental demands exceed a person's perception of their own resources, then high levels of stress will be experienced. Furthermore, if beliefs about effectiveness are pessimistic, then this in turn diminishes motivation, even to try. Most brain-damaged patients have great difficulty in succeeding in almost every aspect of functioning, so reduced motivation is a major extra handicap to be overcome. The constraints of institutions can lead to apathy and create a further barrier against new learning.

A special kind of alienation occurs when people are in hospital. Personal and cultural idiosyncrasies are not so well tolerated as at home, and the patient undergoes a process of deculturalization (Goffman, 1961). When a person has successfully adapted to a hospital life then he loses the special language, shared jokes, gossip and information about the environment from whence he came.

There is also a disruption of family life. Its structure is altered when a member is absent, and reorganization takes place to fill the gap. The new arrangement may be difficult to dismantle when the missing member comes home, especially if the temporary organization suited the needs of the family better than the original. For example, the previous role of wife and mother may not be as satisfactory to a woman as that of 'the head of the household' or 'breadwinner'. Furthermore, responsibilities and obligations are not so pressing while the person is in hospital, and during that time status may be lost so that on discharge the ex-patient may develop a preference for dependence, such as experienced in the unit. Henderson and Parsons (1957) recognized the persuasive nature of the sick role which is easier to adopt in a medical setting because of the cues from the environment. The range of roles is less than outside the unit, so the person adopts the role of 'patient' or 'handicapped'. Both are passive and are valued poorly by society. Some fight against the role initially, so there may be role confusion; i.e. the person does not recognize the 'rules' of being a patient. Sanctions, which are often subconscious, often succeed in moulding the patient into acceptance. Whilst this may ensure a homogeneity of the population, it makes subsequent rehabilitation more difficult.

Finally, and this touches on one of the stages of rehabilitation already referred to, segregation of the physically handicapped from the wider community means that the general public have little chance to become aware of their problems, and of what they have to offer. Thus the stereotype of the handicapped lives on. Only by actively encouraging the handicapped to face the world can the attitudes of society be made more sympathetic and realistic. It is suggested, therefore, that long-term hospital-based rehabilitation service is a contradiction in terms, and makes it less likely that the patient will make maximum physical, mental, vocational, economic and social recovery. The question remains: where, when and how should rehabilitation take place?

5.6 COMMUNITY REHABILITATION

Rehabilitation within the community means that a programme is developed by professionals supplemented where necessary and possible by other carers. These other carers are to be trained and helped and will include the family as most important keyworkers. The team has to capitalize the available resources to be found in the area such as training colleges, schools, adult training schemes, and identify facilities from organizations such as the Manpower Services Commission. The family can be helped as a unit to cope with the stresses involved in long-term rehabilitation. Community rehabilitation is not a complete substitute for inpatient rehabilitation, nor should it be seen as a cheap option to providing residential care, but rather as a better method of using resources, and capable of providing improved care. Conventional outpatient programmes are often uncoordinated, suffer from lack of proper transport, and long periods of waiting and boredom. The development of a community approach was to a considerable extent influenced by Cornwall's geography and its associated transport problems.

5.7 DEVELOPMENT OF THE COMMUNITY REHABILITATION TEAMS (CRTs)

Some years ago a 26 year old Cornishman sustained a severe head injury and was unconscious for approximately 6 weeks. He was transferred from the intensive treatment unit via a surgical ward to the precursor of the CSRU where he received treatment for several months. He made a steady and well documented improvement. Since he had to return home to parents who were pensioners, attempts were made to send him for further residential rehabilitation. A unit out of the county accepted him but found his behaviour unacceptable (he used bad language!) and discharged him. Thereafter no other unit would even consider him. The therapists and social worker who were concerned with his management developed a community-based programme to meet his needs for continuing treatment. It maintains his progress to date (and preserves his parents' sanity).

They arranged first for him to attend a hospital in Truro for hydrotherapy and occupational therapy, another in St Austell for his speech therapy and used his own firm's industrial physiotherapy department. Subsequently they monitored progress and were able to bring in other facilities as needed. This allowed the patient to remain at home and yet receive a full time, integrated programme of rehabilitation. His attendance at hospitals was gradually reduced and he took up sheltered work with his original employers. Even after 4.5 years he has not returned to a high enough standard for open employment but he continues to make progress; and more important, perhaps, he has retained close links with his family and a place in the community (Sapey, 1985).

The group formed the nucleus of the first Cornwall CRT. Over the following 18 months four more CRTs were established. They are geographically placed to cover all the managed areas of Cornwall, and their boundaries are those of Social Services areas.

Membership of the CRTs

All teams have representatives from the district health authority and social services (Table 5.2). Each team has an appointed team leader,

Table 5.2. Representatives on community rehabilitation teams

District health authority
   Consultant in rehabilitation medicine
   Physiotherapist and occupational therapist (from nearest hospital)
   Speech therapist
   Community nurse
   General practitioner, when possible

Social service department
   Social work team leader
   Social worker
   Domiciliary occupational therapist
   Home help organizer

Manpower Services Commission
   Disablement resettlement officer

Jointly funded
   Clinical psychologist
   Social worker in rehabilitation   } (attend all teams)

Occasional attendance, as needed
   Housing officer
   Staff from rehabilitation units

and the venue and secretarial support will come from the office of the leader, whether social services or health authority. The teams meet once a month for 2 hours. A typical agenda will see two or three new patients/clients introduced, and eight or ten others reviewed. Any member of the team can refer a patient, and is responsible for first getting the individual's consent for such discussion. It is specifically explained that information will be shared between the health authority and the social services. The teams deal with most of the conditions which get referred to the rehabilitation service, and each has about ten to twelve patients with brain damage from head injury under review. They will highlight any areas of need and deficiency in service provision, and where deficits are found seek alternatives, then evaluate and check progress.

At the end of each discussion actions are agreed, and the member(s) who are to implement it identified. The official minutes, circulated later serve as an *aide-mémoire*. Progress reports are made at the next meeting. It has a collective role in gathering information about local problems, and potential to act as a local pressure group. They will offer advice and support to each other, to families, other carers, and to the general public, and in the future will act as a focus for research and evaluation.

The CRTs can provide assistance for people already living in the community and for those being discharged from hospitals or the three special rehabilitation facilities. Over the last 3 years 70 patients suffering the effects of severe head injury have been referred to the rehabilitation service. Approximately half have been referred from the hospital service to the CSRU direct. The other half had sustained their injuries previously. For this particular group it has usually been necessary to provide a comprehensive multidisciplinary assessment. For many, this has been the first such assessment provided since their injuries. In the interim they had been coping with extreme difficulty, often without knowledge of help that was in fact readily available. The CRTs can provide a package of treatments which may be concerned with physical or intellectual functioning and identify support services for the individual and those who give them care. This may include use of social clubs, leisure centres, colleges, training facilities, voluntary organizations and other community resources (Evans, 1987).

5.8 CONCLUSION

Community rehabilitation is not to be thought of as a cheap option but as part of a continuum of a rehabilitation service. The CRTs are a forum for professionals who are already in post to meet and exchange views. Such discussions speed decision-making, make best use of available resources and dismantle unhelpful interprofessional barriers. The community approach enables the individual to remain a part of the community while the last stages of rehabilitation are completed. There is less chance that the standards and behaviour of therapists, doctors and social workers will be imposed which, in many situations, can effectively alienate the patient from his original environment.

If the aim is to return the patient to the community then it makes sense to do so as soon as possible. CRTs help in this respect by setting out individual programmes giving more specific treatment than out-patients can usually provide. It is easier to give the family support since there are more people involved who have the whole picture, rather than only a part. For the family it means that an approach to one member of the team can give access to the knowledge of the whole; there is less 'point scoring' between the medical and social services, and there is better understanding of each others' problems and roles. There is much less bureaucracy, decision-making is quicker and there is scope for multidisciplinary research and teaching. Since the patient is at home, family estrangement is less, and the risk of institutionalization is less. The patient (client) can more easily maintain his or her social network and there are fewer transport problems for the family since they do not have to disrupt family life by frequent visits to hospital or rehabilitation unit. There is less chance of isolating the handicapped from their community and this should reduce the chance of encouraging the development of ghettoes of the handicapped.

Back-up is required from residential facilities for programmed care, and crisis relief; there does need to be adequate transport and an enthusiastic integrator. If successful, CRTs allow earlier discharge, and because of better monitoring and better access to scarce resources there is less chance of failed rehabilitation. It is cheaper than residential care, but this should not be an aim. Rather it must be argued that this will help to redress the inadequacies of our present services to this group of handicapped people.

REFERENCES

Abramson, P.D., Seligman, M. and Teasdale, G. (1978) Learned helplessness in humans. *J. Abnorm. Psychiat.*, **87**, 49–74.

Bryden, J., *Community Prevalence of Post Head Injury Disability*, in preparation.

Evans, C.D. (1987) Community Rehabilitation. *Clinical Rehabilitation*, Edward Arnold, London.

Freidson, E. (1975) *The Profession of Medicine*, Dodd Mead Co., New York.

Goffman, E. (1961) *Asylums. Essays on the Social Status of Mental Patients and Inmates*, Penguin, Harmondsworth.

Harrison, J. (1986) *The Young Disabled Adult*, Royal College of Physicians, London.

Henderson, A.M. and Parsons, T. (1957) *Theory of Social and Economic Organisations*, Free Press, New York.

Illich, I. (1977) *Limits to Medicine*, Penguin, Harmondsworth.

Kennedy, I. (1980) The Reith Lectures: *Style, Responsibility and Accountability. Brit. Med. J.*, **281**, 6256–58.

Lazarus, R.S. and Monat, A. (eds) (1977) *Stress and Coping: an anthology*, Columbia University Press, New York.

London, P.S. (Chairman) (1987) Report of a Steering Committee: *A Rehabilitation Service for the West Midlands*, West Midlands Regional Health Authority.

Sapey, R.S. (1985) Tailor-made Rehabilitation. *Social Work Today*, July, pp. 18–19.

Wade, D. and Langton Hewer, R. (1987) Epidemiology of some neurological conditions with specific reference to the work load on the NHS. *Int. Rehabil. Med.*, **8**, 129–37.

Zola, I. (1977) *The Disabling Professions*, I. Illich (ed.), Marian Boyars, London.

PART THREE

Models of treatment

6   A salient factors approach to brain injury rehabilitation

Rodger Ll. Wood

There has been a recognizable attempt over the past 8 years to make brain injury rehabilitation a distinct and specialized service in rehabilitation medicine. Before 1980 most brain injury rehabilitation centres provided treatment based on principles of general (physical) rehabilitation medicine, adopting the practices and organizational methods inherent in that traditional rehabilitation model. This meant that treatment tended to be directed by the physician and orientated according to the treatment of goals of individual disciplines. These goals were often determined by criteria which emphasized physical recovery from injury, and this became the main index by which the outcome of rehabilitation was measured. Gradually, it became clear that this traditional model was not appropriate for brain injury rehabilitation. The reasons for this are largely based on the nature of the recovery process, the diversity of rehabilitation needs, and the fact that character changes, which are unique to brain injury, alter certain aspects of behaviour and affect the way brain-injured individuals cope with the demands of community living.

6.1 UNDERSTANDING RECOVERY

The brain injury rehabilitation community has been slow to acquire information that will help guide approaches to treatment planning, predicting patterns of recovery or the response of certain groups of patients to particular rehabilitation techniques. For example, the speed, pattern and extent of recovery can vary according to the nature of the injury (Hall and Cope, 1985). The most rapid period of recovery takes place during the first 12 to 24 months and many of the changes that take place during this time have a spontaneous quality.

Rehabilitation during this period is still necessary, however, in order to facilitate or expedite the recovery process and prevent complications developing. The nature of the brain injury can also determine the quality of outcome. Some types of brain damage are associated with a poorer prognosis for recovery than others; e.g. frontal or brain-stem injury following head trauma has been associated with long-term disability, poor social adjustment, and a failure to successfully re-integrate back into the community (Thomsen, 1984). The type of brain damage produced by Herpes simplex encephalitis also carries a poor prognosis because it frequently results in a dense amnesic condition that does not seem to improve over time or significantly respond to specific forms of therapy.

Recovery from brain injury also depends on the quality, intensity and duration of rehabilitation. Hall and Cope (1985) point out that there has been a lack of rigorous scientific assessment of rehabilitation techniques and, as was suggested in Chapter 3, it is not clear which elements of rehabilitation are instrumental to recovery and which are incidental. The lack of research on the actual process of rehabilitation means that little hard data is available to help the clinicians decide how much, or what kind of treatment should be provided, or when. Consequently, patients tend to receive all available forms of therapy from the time rehabilitation begins. It may be however, that for some types of disability or following certain types of brain damage, therapy resources should in introduced gradually and selectively, rather than en masse, thus avoiding the practice of treatment according to availability rather than treatment by design!

We know that there are different stages in the recovery process, with physical recovery generally proceeding at a rate which is faster than cognitive recovery (Bond and Brooks, 1976; Mackworth and Cope, 1982). There may be some merit therefore, in a technique which introduces different types of therapy at a time when they are likely to exert a maximum effect. This would require a more precise knowledge of the recovery process from different types of injury than currently exists, but a more selective application of therapy might result in considerable savings in the cost of rehabilitation because of reductions in staff time.

A 'salient factors' approach to brain injury rehabilitation is designed to provide an operational framework that can help rehabilitation professionals organize their thinking in respect of how the treatment they provide relates to the nature of the brain injury and pattern of disability. It tries to offer a more individualized approach to brain injury rehabilitation, using procedures and practices that make medical or clinical sense, and which lend themselves to scientific evaluation.

The essence of a salient factors approach is to understand the organic basis of social and physical handicap. It assumes that a knowledge of the origins of the clinical disability, in relation to the brain damage sustained, will help in the planning of rehabilitation. Treatment plans are formulated by combining relevant clinical and psychosocial factors; the former describing how the injury contributes to the patient's current condition; the latter indicating the type of environment to which the patient may return, which may have implications for both the type, and goals of therapy. As such, the clinical and psychosocial data provide sets of information which can influence the actual treatment process, the latter establishing a framework and a purpose for the former by specifying the potential goals of treatment. In turn, this can determine how treatment priorities should be assessed. Any treatment plan will need to address short-, medium- and long-term objectives, and should take into account the spontaneous process of recovery and the patient's changing needs as recovery continues.

The approach demands a change in the attitude of therapy staff rather than any change in rehabilitation techniques *per se*. This is because it is the way that rehabilitation is organized, rather than the type of rehabilitation given, that is likely to lead to a successful treatment outcome. Implicit in this approach is an interdisciplinary way of working, in order to promote communication between therapy staff and increase the cohesiveness of a treatment team. It is perhaps important to emphasize that the team must include nurses, as well as therapists, if one seeks to provide better continuity of patient care.

6.2 SALIENT FACTORS INFLUENCING BRAIN INJURY REHABILITATION

Table 6.1 shows the three major categories (organic, psychosocial and treatment) that combine to form the salient factors approach. As

Table 6.1 Salient factors of brain injury rehabilitation

Organic factors	Psychosocial factors	Treatment factors
Injury characteristics	Pre-accident characteristics	Organization of treatment team
Measures of severity	Family dynamics	Generation of training
Pattern of disability	Potential for employment	Evaluating and reporting progress
Identifying clinical 'constraints'		

stated above, the injury characteristics and a person's psychosocial system contain information which should help a rehabilitation team properly evaluate the treatment priorities in relation to potential discharge goals. **Treatment factors** exist as a product of categories 1 and 2 and actually describe the 'ingredients' of the treatment process.

The need to evaluate all these factors and combine them into an approach (or model) for organizing treatment may seem obvious to some rehabilitation professionals, but many rehabilitation teams seem to give little thought to the actual brain injury itself. This usually leads to a lack of attention to the organic basis for the residual pattern of brain damage, reducing the chances of recognizing organically determined disorders of behaviour or learning disability. The salient factors approach, by providing a comprehensive picture of the dynamics of the injury and how they interact with the personal, social and treatment history of the patient, can help the rehabilitation team 'fine tune' their treatment methods according to a patient's pattern of disability, without overlooking how the brain injury interacts with the observed clinical abnormalities. It is assumed that an awareness of these salient factors will play a major role in the success or failure of a rehabilitation plan by differentially guiding the attention of the treatment team to pertinent clinical characteristics that help determine priorities of treatment.

Organic factors

Characteristics of injury

Jennett and Teasdale (1981) suggest that very often, a narrow interpretation of brain injury is adopted, based on a certain 'clinicopathological type'. They advise that in order to understand properly the characteristics of the brain injury, clinical staff need to be able to answer the following questions:

1. How did the injury occur?
2. What are the clinical measures of severity?
3. What structural or dynamic pathology has taken place in the brain?

In the case of head injury for example, the brain can be damaged by structural disruption and distortion, metabolic or anoxic changes or, as is most usually the case, by a combination of these pathological processes. Jennett and Teasdale state that the basic mechanisms producing brain damage are fairly well understood. What is not clear, however, is the relationship of specific types of damage or mechanisms of injury to the outcome of rehabilitation.

Knowledge of the type of injury, the mechanism of injury and the presence or absence of secondary complications, may explain the nature of an individual's physical, cognitive or emotional state. With sufficient clinical experience, these facts may allow a prediction of how a patient, with a certain pattern of deficits in relation to certain types of injury, will respond to treatment. This would be an important step in assessing an individual's potential for rehabilitation and would also help rehabilitation staff gauge their own expectations of a patient's progress in therapy.

The majority of professionals who work with the brain-injured have rejected the **unitary concept** of brain damage (Walsh, 1978). However, it is still not clear how many rehabilitation professionals fully understand the diversity of the brain injuries they deal with. Knowledge of the type of injury, location of primary damage, and mechanisms involved in the production of injury, can assist the rehabilitation team in predicting treatment needs and patterns of recovery. For example, the label 'head injury' is not a sufficient definition for the understanding of that category of brain damage because the dynamics of head injury vary according to the circumstances of that injury. A motor vehicle accident usually involves acceleration/deceleration forces which cause the brain to move within the skull cavity, producing a diffuse pattern of damage. Even so, the extent of the damage depends on such factors as velocity of head movement, presence or absence of skull fracture, haematomas or haemorrhagic contusions, raised intracranial pressure, or the presence of anoxia. Head injuries which do not include deceleration factors (such as some sporting injuries, assaults with a blunt instrument, or having a stone fall on one's head) will not involve the same energy distribution effects and therefore, exert less of a concussive force, producing a more localized injury. When the injury includes a fracture of the skull casing there is an increased risk of complications such as meningitis or epilepsy (especially when skull fragments penetrate the dura mater). If these complications can be avoided, however, the actual fracturing of the skull casing can ironically have some beneficial effects, because the fracture takes much of the force out of the impact, reducing the more general concussive effects of the injury.

Perhaps the major distinction between brain injuries which do not involve deceleration forces compared to those which do, is the extent to which the frontal and brain stem structures are involved. Individuals with frontal injury display many alterations of personality and character, in particular, diminished insight and a lack of social awareness. This means that whatever the extent of their physical recovery, the social handicaps which remain may prevent them from utilizing these physical abilities to their full advantage. Alternatively, individuals who have primarily sustained a brain stem injury, suffer from severe physical deficits. These often exist in the context of well preserved intellectual ability which is 'locked-in' because the person cannot express himself, either verbally or by gesture. Other brain injuries, such as stroke, encephalitis or low velocity missile wounds, involve different mechanisms (both to head injury and each other) all of which directly or indirectly influence the pattern of clinical abnormalities.

The value of identifying the mechanism of injury may be assessed by whether or not this leads to better predictions of outcome or a recognition that certain types of injury produce particular patterns of disability. It is clear that a serious brain injury may be sustained without necessarily producing serious consequences. By relating type of injury to consequences of injury, we may become better at predicting response to treatment, or even what treatment to give and when; thereby reducing costs of health care and improving effectiveness of treatment.

Indices of brain damage

When trying to establish the pattern of injury, it is important to obtain as many objective indices of damage as possible. At present, objective clinical indices are determined by neuroradiological investigations, electroencephalograph (EEG) records or evoked responses. However, these sophisticated methods cannot always be relied upon to provide corroborative evidence of clinical abnormalities. A recent study by Groswasser et al. (1987) reported that 11 out of 130 severe concussional injuries had normal computerized tomography (CT) scans. Lipper et al. (1985) also commented on a discrepancy between normal CT scans and a wide variety of neurobehavioural findings, such as memory disturbance and subjective complaints of headaches and dizziness. The Groswasser et al. study showed that MRI scans were far more sensitive than CT scans in demonstrating residual post-traumatic brain lesions. Patients with persistent neurobehavioural disturbances, whose CT scans did not contribute evidence of brain injury following severe concussion, were investigated using the higher resolution MRI scan. Groswasser et al. found that the MRI scans indicated damage to the frontal and temporal lobes, as would be predicted by Courville's findings (Courville, 1943). Groswasser and his colleagues argue that knowledge of the nature of the brain injury allows a 'better understanding of the patient's clinical and neurobehavioural disturbances.'

Caution must also be applied when dealing with EEG data. Jennett and Teasdale (1981), describing the development of late onset epilepsy in persons who have sustained severe brain injury, comment that 'some 20% of patients who subsequently develop late epilepsy, have a normal EEG in the early stages after injury'. Another study by Jabbari et al. (1986) on 515 Vietnam veterans who sustained penetrating missile wounds, found that 46% had normal EEGs and 11% displayed an EEG pattern of 'unknown clinical significance'. EEGs are therefore not reliable indicators of organically determined disorders of behaviour, especially when mood changes or sudden unexplained outbursts are observed. When such a behaviour pattern is present, treatment staff should seek expert advice on the patient's EEG to discover whether volatile changes of mood and temperament, or variable levels of alertness and awareness which cannot be attributed to changes in medication or fatigue, may have 'electrical' origins.

The problem in obtaining an 'expert' opinion is that there do not appear to be many 'experts' available who can recognize EEG patterns which are not typical of classical epilepsy. Data is currently being collected (Wood, in preparation) on a series of patients with episodic mood changes and associated behaviour disorders, who have received standard EEG investigations. So far, there seems to be a total lack of correlation between the EEG record and the clearly observed pattern of neurobehavioural abnormalities. After serious head injury, many EEG records have an atypical quality (as in the study by Jabbari et al., 1986) which may suggest temporal lobe abnormalities, or **limbic epilepsy** – the kind associated with behaviour and cognitive changes, yet formal confirmation of an organic basis for the behaviour cannot be obtained. In this respect the comment of Teuber (1969) is apt, 'absence of evidence is not evidence of absence', and this may be the best rule of thumb when considering the origin of many emotional and behavioural problems!

Assessing the nature of disability

Any assessment in rehabilitation should try to associate observed abnormalities, or recorded impairment, with the patient's injury characteristics, in case these prove to have some predictive value for rehabilitation outcome. Such an attempt at associating types of brain injury with patterns of disability may at least allow the growth of information concerning how mechanisms of brain injury and patterns of damage respond to different forms of treatment. The nature of the assessment process in rehabilitation is coming under increasing scrutiny. Hart and Hayden (1985), Lezack (1987) and Wood (1987a) have all commented on the lack of correspondence between test data and the functional deficits which are the 'stuff' of rehabilitation. Sarno (1985) argued this point in relation to an assessment of speech disorders. She stated that:

> Rehabilitation evaluations must incorporate observations of the aphasic in his natural environment as part of the overall communication assessment by using a functional communication measure. In other words, communication must go beyond the restricted information derived from standardised language tests. (Sarno, 1985, p. 167)

The traditional neuropsychological assessment has come under similar criticism. Hart and Hayden (1985) argue for greater 'ecological value' in assessment procedures used for rehabilitation. They maintain that measures of outcome are of little value if all they demonstrate is a change on some clinical measure which is irrelevant to the everyday functioning of the patient:

> Clinicians experienced with head injury are painfully aware that many of these patients function essentially within normal limits on many formal neuropsychological tests and then show significant difficulties at work, in social situations or at school.
> (Hart and Hayden, 1985, p. 206)

This argument was echoed by Wood (1987a) and has also been used as an argument for a more functionally oriented approach to assessment by Diller and Gordon (1981). In essence, whatever the problem being evaluated or the discipline of the examiner, information must be provided which is meaningful in terms of what the treatment team must achieve to produce a good recovery. If the content of a professional report in rehabilitation does not directly inform the treatment team how to organize their therapy towards a specific treatment goal, then the report is lacking in substance and clinical utility.

Abrams et al. (1973) argued that because medical progress is often dependent upon psychosocial factors, such factors deserve the same precise, objective terminology, and objective standards that are given to medical conditions. This argument cannot be denied and will receive further attention later but, for the moment, these remarks point to another weakness in the evaluation of the legacies of brain injury – the terminology used to describe the condition of the patient.

Several authors have commented on the confused terminology of the legacies of brain injury (e.g. Duckworth, 1983; Wood, 1987a). In Chapter 12 of this book Haffey and Johnson also comment on this and present a model for evaluating the outcome of rehabilitation using clearly defined terms, distinguishing between 'impairment', 'disability' and 'handicap'. The reason for introducing terminology in a section on treatment approaches is that specific treatment techniques and goals of therapy are influenced by the words we use to describe the abnormalities displayed by patients.

In rehabilitation there has been an abuse of the word 'impairment'. Diller and Gordon (1981) cautioned against a too liberal use of this term and question whether impairment or the products of impairment should be the focus of rehabilitation (the products of impairment being disability and social handicap). Granger (1983) argued that individuals with even serious impairment need not experience an equal degree of social handicap, if the proper balance between attitude, motivation and social supports can be developed. Diller and Gordon (1981) point out that an impairment (such as a lost limb) can mean different things to different people depending on how such impairment interferes with their lifestyle. Newcombe (1981) reported how one of her patients, a surgeon who has sustained a missile wound, continued to display a marked impairment on visuospatial tasks during neuropsychological assessment, without any comparable effect on his behaviour or visuomotor skills as a practicing surgeon.

Duckworth (1983) recommends that the disability which follows injury should be described in terms of behaviour. Stolov (1982) also felt that this would be a more meaningful way to describe disability and emphasized the loss of social, vocational and psychological function, as well as physical function. In his review of this problem Duckworth concluded that when conceived in this way rehabilitation becomes more the correction of deviance from social norms than the correction of malfunction alone.

By encouraging members of a clinical team to describe the legacies of injury in terms of their behavioural manifestations, it becomes easier to identify realistic treatment goals which are relevant targets for all members of the clinical team. This avoids compartmentalizing the patient according to different therapy categories and treatment approaches. It also helps prevent treatment being applied in a fragmented and discipline-bound way because when the target of rehabilitation is formulated in terms of behaviour, all members of the treatment team can integrate their efforts to achieve a common goal. The progress to this goal can then be objectively evaluated, according to behavioural criteria and single-case study methods (see Goldstein, 1983).

The salient factors approach to an evaluation of the legacies of injury emphasizes the way brain injury has disrupted a person's 'lifestyle'. This means that disability is related more to social handicap than impairment, and treatment is directed more towards re-establishing a way of life for the patient than correcting 'clinical' abnormalities that may have no real-life significance.

Clinical constraints

A clinical constraint is something which acts as an obstacle to the treatment process. The two main forms of constraint upon the process of rehabilitation are inappropriate administration of drugs and the reduced capacity for information processing and attention imposed by the injury.

1. Medication. Progress in rehabilitation depends upon how well a patient learns techniques to overcome disability. Learning is influenced by arousal, and an awareness of social or environmental cues which influence behaviour change. Drugs which reduce arousal, or alter a person's level of awareness will inevitably have an adverse effect upon learning ability and progress in rehabilitation. In Chapter 10 Eames discussed 'abuses' of medication in some detail. The purpose of including a comment here is to point out the specific ways in which these **iatrogenic** effects of medication operate.

Thompson and Trimble (1982) reported on the influence of anti-epileptic drugs such as phenobarbitone, phenytoin, sodium valproate and carbamazepine on a range of cognitive functions. It was found that phenobarbitone and phenytoin in particular had a marked depressant effect on cognitive functions, slowing down the rate of information processing, and potentially elevating the individual's confused state. These studies were done on normal subjects and it is probable that, following brain injury, the detrimental influence of these drugs is increased significantly, interfering with attention and concentration and, by implication, many aspects of learning and memory.

The usual justification for anticonvulsants in the absence of epileptic abnormalities is to prevent epilepsy from occurring. There is some question however, about whether or not the prophylactic use of anticonvulsants is justified (McQueen *et al.*, 1983), especially when one considers the way these drugs affect other aspects of recovery, and a patient's response to rehabilitation. In a review of the management of post-traumatic epilepsy Willmore (1985) concluded that there is no support for the hypothesis that phenytoin administration will prevent the development of post-traumatic epilepsy.

The use of sedative drugs to control abusive, aggressive or threatening behaviour is also open to criticism. Clinical experience has shown that when such medication is prescribed for brain-injured patients it is usually administered in small doses. This dosage is rarely sufficient to act as a 'chemical straight jacket' and, in many cases, the medication produces even greater confusion and an agitated manner. In such circumstances the patient's awareness of the consequences of his or her behaviour is reduced and therefore he or she is less amenable to social influences, and less capable of learning by experience.

Another criticism of sedatives involves the action of different groups of drugs on the central nervous system. Drugs of the phenothiazine groups have an epileptogenic quality. They may precipitate late onset epilepsy and even exacerbate mood changes (and their accompanying behaviour disorders) if these mood states have their origins in some form of abnormal electrical activity. In some cases, this could mean that the medication will make the patient's condition worse rather than better.

For less severe cases of agitated or difficult behaviour, tranquilizing medication is often prescribed, using drugs from the benzodiazepine group. The majority of these drugs contain an anxziolytic component which will reduce an individual's level of anxiety and may enhance the disinhibited quality of behaviour. For patients who have sustained frontal damage, and therefore display behaviour which is already rather disinhibited and poorly controlled, the introduction of valium or similar drugs may only serve to exacerbate the behaviour problem and, again, interfere with social learning and the development of appropriate emotional self-control.

2. *Attention deficits.* The other major clinical constraint is not imposed by inappropriate medical intervention but by a failure to recognize the role of certain neuropsychological mechanisms which are important for learning. Progress in rehabilitation is inevitably affected when the apparatus which mediates learning (the cortex and certain mid-brain structures) is damaged. The single most important system mediating learning and memory is the **information processing system.** It is this system which regulates the passage of information throughout the brain and determines the individual's ability to focus or sustain attention, and the speed at which he can monitor, organize and respond to information.

The relationship between the information processing system, learning and memory has long been acknowledged (Posner and Boies, 1971) and Wood (1987b) argues that many aspects of behaviour important to brain injury rehabilitation depend on an intact information processsing system. However, this neuropsychological system is very vulnerable to the concussional forces which operate during head injury, and attentional deficits are among the most prominent and long-lasting cognitive disturbances associated with concussional damage to the brain. This has obvious implications for rehabilitation. In order to benefit from almost any form of therapy, a patient has to sit and listen to the instructions given by the therapist; a process which requires considerable information processing capability, involving attention span, attention capacity, and memory.

Discrimination-learning studies have shown that attentional deficits prevent many head-injured patients focusing on a training task, making it difficult to select the salient characteristics of the task from the complex array of information available (Wood, 1987b). Attentional factors were found to be more important than intellectual ability (measured by standardized tests) as far as speed of learning was concerned. Neuropsychological, and other cognitive forms of assessment, should therefore attempt to define how well a patient can attend in therapy sessions and how much of the information presented to them is properly understood. This implies that treatment approaches should be sufficiently flexible in order to accommodate a patient's limited information processing ability and not impose learning strategies or information sets which are too complex for the patient to easily understand and respond to.

Psychosocial factors

The success of rehabilitation depends not only on the organization of treatment but also the quality and amount of family support available. Abrams, Neville and Becker (1973) felt that the impact of psychosocial, vocational and educational problems on medical progress can be so profound that their evaluation should be considered a fundamental part of the data collection leading to rehabilitation planning.

Few rehabilitation professionals are unaware of the burden experienced by a family trying to cope with an individual who is both physically handicapped and mentally impaired. The work of Brooks and McKinlay (1983); Oddy, Humphrey and Uttley (1978), and the long-term follow-up studies of Thomsen in Denmark (Thomsen, 1984) indicate the need to consider social factors as a major part of the rehabilitation process. In many cases, however, there seems to be a dislocation in the thinking of treatment staff concerning their attitude to the social factors that prevail in rehabilitation setting. On the one hand, they acknowledge the importance of the family and the need for appropriate discharge planning but, on the other hand, fail to design an individual's rehabilitation programme so that the goals of therapy reflect meaningful social issues which may actually have implications for treatment itself. Some factors are central to the process of rehabilitation, such as the attitudes that a patient brings to the rehabilitation setting or the degree of support that can be expected from the patient's family. These factors are considered more fully below.

Pre-accident characteristics

Some assessments of a patient's pre-accident personality and family relationships can be extremely important in assessing how an individual is likely to react in a rehabilitation setting. Brain injury upsets the balance of many personality characteristics, causing disinhibited behaviour. This means that character traits which were present before the brain injury may be exacerbated in a way which appears disproportionate to the rest of behaviour, or the individual's emotional disposition. It is not uncommon to find that patients who are rigid and autocratic in a treatment setting have a pre-accident history of such behaviour. This is not meant to imply that their pre-accident behaviour was pathological in any way, but it does suggest that personality characteristics that were considered acceptable before injury take on a different flavour after injury. For example, a rather methodical person may develop a rigid, obsessional style of thinking and behaving; an individual with an assertive manner may become domineering or even aggressive; while a rather superficial person, who may have led a fairly dissolute lifestyle, comes to display behaviour or personality characteristics that have almost a sociopathic quality.

It has been argued by Abrams *et al.* (1973) that the treatment team should possess as much knowledge as possible about pre-injury behaviour in order to have realistic expectations about the degree of motivation that is likely to be displayed by the patient. This will affect the type of cooperation that may be obtained, his observance of medically prescribed routines, his social values, attitudes to authority, level of self-control, and a host of other social refinements that are expected in a professional interaction of this kind. Premorbid characteristics represent the 'fabric' of behaviour and are therefore the 'material' that therapy staff have to work with. It is unlikely, therefore, that a treatment team would be able to turn a person with a dubious pre-accident character, possibly including alcohol or drug abuse and some form of antisocial conduct, into a virtuous, socially disciplined individual (especially if frontal damage is part of the clinical picture).

Studies by Jamieson and Kelly (1973) reported by Bond (1984) suggest that many victims of head injury have premorbid personal or social characteristics which predispose them to injury. Basically, these include immature personality and an impulsive style of behaviour. It would, of course, be a vast over-generalization to say that the majority of those who sustain brain injury in motor vehicle accidents have dubious social histories, but it is a fact that a significant number of car accidents are the result of 'drunken driving'. This implies an immature,

or irresponsible attitude that is not going to be improved by
\jury. Individuals with this kind of personality can adversely
...fluence the therapist-patient relationship. Because this can alter the
expectations of treatment outcome it is important that the presence of
such characteristics should not be overlooked.

In addition to personality factors, the presence of subtle
developmental anomalies should be considered. It is surprising how
many individuals who sustain head injury report a history of learning
difficulties (best described as dyslexia). These characteristics are often
revealed by neuropsychological assessment post-injury. Before the
accident individuals with these developmental anomalies experienced
difficulty focusing and maintaining a level of attention, organizing
thinking, or sequentially ordering responses. These pre-accident
cognitive anomalies will inevitably influence attentiveness and learning
ability in a rehabilitation setting.

Family dynamics and the treatment process

Family members bring a set of attitudes to a clinical setting which may
be at considerable variance from those possessed by experienced
rehabilitation staff. Relatives may assume that treatment (of any kind)
will lead to a 'cure' or a resumption of the quality and style of
behaviour they have always associated with their relative. The gradual
realization by family members that many of their expectations are not
going to be fulfilled can precipitate a feeling of resentment towards the
treatment team. This usually manifests itself as an attitude of distrust,
with a number of criticisms being made about the quality or quantity
of treatment provided for their relative. Although some of these
criticisms may be justified, the majority are most likely a reflection of
grief and a state of agitation by the relative over their inability to
control the healing process and obtain a 'cure'.

The tension experienced by the family at this time will exacerbate any
intrafamily conflicts which may have existed before the accident and
create new ones. A spouse who may have shared a close, supportive
and loving relationship with the person before the accident now finds
it difficult to adjust to accommodate changes in their partner's behaviour.
Relationships between a child and an injured parent may also be seriously
strained once the child realizes how the pre-accident family hierarchy
has changed, with the parent now dependent upon the child instead
of the other way round. This is particularly difficult when the child is
a young adolescent. Such changes in family dynamics have important
implications in deciding how discharge goals should be formulated and
what role the family should have in the rehabilitation process.

Once factors such as family expectations and patient aspirations are determined, the treatment team can plan therapy accordingly and provide the family with a clear understanding about the intermediate and long-term treatment objectives. This in turn provides the family with an opportunity for becoming involved with some of the goals of therapy, allowing them to have a feeling of control over the recovery process, helping them adjust to the different types of impairment displayed by the patient. Family involvement offers the treatment team an opportunity to train individual family members to deal with problems or difficulties generated by the brain-injured relative. It is important to realize that these 'social factors' are not extrinsic to treatment, but are central to the success of rehabilitation and should be included as an element of every treatment plan.

Equally important to the attitudes and expectations of the family are the expectations of the patient, because the protracted nature of the recovery process is bound to lead to a feeling of disillusionment and a degree of helplessness which may precipitate a depressive reaction or a state of apathy (Seligman, 1975). If there is a chance that such a psychological reaction has occurred then it is the task of the rehabilitation team to identify it and include, as part of therapy, methods which will alleviate that reaction, probably by setting rehabilitation goals that are reasonably easy to achieve and thus provide motivation to achieve other goals.

Potential for education and employment

The ultimate goal of many individuals who receive rehabilitation is not only to return to the community but also to regain some form of employment. It has become evident that the employability of many individuals who have sustained brain injury is greatly influenced, not only by their pre-accident personalities, but also educational and occupational experience. Dresser et al. (1973) found that pre-injury mental status was the single most important factor predicting the employability of 864 Korean war veterans who sustained head injury. She reviewed studies linking re-employment and education in the head-injured and these confirmed the importance of pre-injury educational level in returning to work, especially in those who were mildly injured.

Brain injury survivors who have modest qualifications or work experience limited to factory or unskilled areas of employment are, in many cases, less motivated to return to work but, in principle, are no less employable than individuals who have high school or college backgrounds and managerial or professional experience. The advantage

viduals with a managerial background (especially if they were
large organization) is that work of a less technical or complex
ay be made available, allowing the individual to retain their
onal identity by remaining part of their familiar organizational
system. There are probably more options available to 'white collar'
workers because the majority have a greater range of work experience
than unskilled manual workers. Also many clerical types of employment are better suited to individuals with physical handicap, for whom
a sedentary lifestyle would be acceptable.

It is not necessarily the case, however, that academic achievement
or a management background will increase the chances of successful
employment. Many individuals are not prepared to accept what they
perceive as a 'lower' form of occupation, compared to the one they
enjoyed before the accident. A bank manager for example, may not
be prepared to accept a job as a clerical worker because he is not able
to make the kind of personal adjustment that accompanies such a
change in role. Similarly, people with clerical or administrative
backgrounds may find it difficult to transfer to assembly tasks or other
forms of factory work because this involves repetitive and probably
boring routines of work.

The task of the rehabilitation team is to assess an individual's potential for employment (at any level) and then include the social and
functional skills appropriate to that employment as part of the retraining programme. Later in rehabilitation some vocational training
should be offered but many aspects of *work behaviour* are just as important as technical ability when it comes to holding down a job and
these characteristics can be a target of therapy from quite early on in
the rehabilitation process. The need to improve attention to task,
accuracy and reliability in following instructions, maintaining a plea-
sant social manner, and possessing a reliable memory, are all factors
which are important in a work setting. These can be included as
targets for therapy just as soon as the treatment team recognize the
individual's potential for re-employment.

Treatment factors

Rehabilitative procedures need to be based upon a careful evaluation
of the organic, clinical and psychosocial factors referred to in the
earlier sections of this chapter. This may seem an absurdly simple
point to make but many rehabilitation centres seem unaware of how
both the process and outcome of rehabilitation can be determined by
certain 'salient factors' which should be identified before treatment
planning takes place. These 'salient factors' may help clarify the goals

of the rehabilitation team, according to the predicted pattern or rate of recovery associated with the injury, as well as the type of person receiving treatment, the attitudes of the family, and the occupational or wider social support system to which the patient is destined to return.

Some general guidelines should be considered during treatment planning:

1. Different types of injuries produce different patterns of disabilities and rates of recovery. Knowledge of the type of injury could help determine treatment priorities;
2. Treatment should be 'outcome oriented', rather than 'discipline oriented'. This means that it is directed towards reducing social handicap, adopting behavioural criteria for measuring treatment effectiveness;
3. Treatment goals should reflect a patient's potential level of recovery and capacity for independence (a judgement based on the experience of the treatment team). Treatment should be directed at improving *behaviour*, as it relates to social and functional skills. This focus for rehabilitation should prevent the narrow and compartmentalized thinking that often results in *clinical progress* being made, but without corresponding *functional independence* being achieved;
4. Targets for therapy are established on the basis of short, intermediate and long-term goals. Short-term goals can be considered to be the priorities of treatment. They usually comprise some aspect of disability or behaviour which, if not improved, becomes a major obstacle preventing other aspects of rehabilitation training. Treatment priorities are often labour intensive and therefore, it is unlikely that a treatment team can address more than three at a time;
5. Intermediate and long-term goals of treatment can be addressed at the same time as short-term priorities but the efforts of the treatment team are likely to be less intensive than would be the case with treatment priorities. A 'lower profile' of training should not, however, be construed as an absence of training or as a reduction in the significance or importance of these goals. Longer-term goals are more closely identified with the discharge goals and hopefully are achieved as a result of evolution in the process of recovery;
6. Continuous evaluation of treatment should be undertaken, using single case methodology and behavioural criteria as a basis for evaluating clinical progress.

To ensure an optimal response from therapy staff as well as the patient, it is important that treatment be organized in such a way that continuity of therapy input is assured. This depends on:

1. communication between treatment staff about the goals of treatment being maintained;
2. an intra (or trans) disciplinary approach being applied;
3. progress made in the clinic becoming generalized to the community, and consolidated there before rehabilitation is stopped;
4. methods adopted which evaluate response to treatment and report functional change to families, as well as referring or funding agencies.

A system of management is required for such a diverse treatment process. Experience has shown that one member of the treatment team should be designated clinical coordinator. This person should adopt a long-term perspective, keeping track of all treatment activities, helping staff maintain a focus upon designated discharge goals. This perspective should also be sufficiently flexible to allow consideration of how factors peripheral to treatment may actually impact upon treatment. This role is probably best filled by the physician or neuropsychologist because, theoretically, by virtue of their training, they are most able to integrate all the available information into a plan for treatment. This is not always the case of course, and there is no necessity for the coordinator's role to be restricted to these disciplines. One can find therapy professionals from a number of disciplines who are more than able to fulfil the coordinator's role.

Organization of the treatment team

1. Communication. Getting treatment staff to talk to one another is one of the most difficult tasks for any clinical coordinator! Therapists report what they are doing but they rarely welcome (or take) advice from colleagues of other disciplines, neither do they readily present information about their treatment methods that invites evaluation or constructive criticism. Until quite recently it was not unusual to find that one therapy discipline in a treatment team did not know (and probably did not care) what the treatment goals of colleagues in other therapy disciplines were.

When this type of interpersonal environment prevails it tends to result in a 'diluted' treatment process, with therapists working in parallel, rather than coordinating their efforts and focussing them upon a common treatment goal. For example, a physical therapist may be concentrating on leg strengthening exercises in order to reduce the disability produced by hemiplegia. At the same time the nursing staff may be struggling to assist the patient on and off the toilet. The efforts of the two groups should therefore be coordinated to achieve the same functional goal which comprises mobility training directed towards some functional goal.

2. *Interdisciplinary.* Following on from communication is the obvious problem of how staff are organized to work together. Eames (Chapter 4) has urged the importance of an interdisciplinary approach to rehabilitation. This attitude has been echoed by a number of rehabilitation professionals and the intention of raising this point again is not to reiterate the argument as such, but to confront individuals with the distinction between 'multidisciplinary' and 'inter-disciplinary' and what they mean in clinical practice.

The essence of an interdisciplinary approach is that therapists actually overlap in the work they do and share responsibility for reaching specific treatment goals, which may have a multidisciplinary significance. However, unless one has worked in a truly inter-disciplinary environment it is difficult to appreciate the advantages it offers. One typical example occurred in the case of the patient being treated at the Kemsley Unit, Northampton, UK, where an inter-disciplinary style of working has been adopted.

The patient had a brain-stem injury and needed speech training to improve articulation and verbal communication. However, the patient did not have a good relationship with the speech therapist. This was partly because the patient was poorly motivated (a constraint imposed by the brain injury) but also, the personality and style of behaviour of the patient conflicted with that of the therapist, and a major breakdown in relationship ensued. Fortunately, this patient did have a good relationship with the physiotherapists. It was therefore decided to try and avoid the interpersonal *impasse* that was preventing therapy. This was achieved by stopping speech training *per se* and increasing the amount of contact with the physiotherapists. The purpose of this was to allow the physiotherapists to include, informally and casually, some of the strategies for speech training that had been devised by the speech therapist. This meant that the speech therapist advised the physiotherapist on what to expect (in terms of articulation) from the patient, and suggested ways in which clarity of speech could be obtained.

In the course of verbally interacting with the patient during physical therapy exercises (according to a prescribed procedure devised by the speech therapist), the physiotherapist subtly trained the patient to improve articulation. The training method was continued until it became a habit for the patient to use that particular strategy for verbal expression. As such, the patient was given all the physical therapy that was required, plus a successful speech therapy programme, without staff having to cope with unmotivated or antagonistic behaviour from the patient towards a particular member of staff.

This is only one example of the flexibility offered by the inter-disciplinary way of working. Other advantages include combining expertise from different therapy disciplines in the treatment of a patient (therapists working together to produce the degree of change that could not be obtained if each therapy was administered separately). More importantly it includes the use of nursing staff as primary therapists. Nurses are available for longer periods of time than therapy staff and can be trained to implement many rehabilitation procedures, under supervision from appropriate therapists. In many ways, the use of nursing in a rehabilitation role offers an ideal and cost-effective way of extending the amount of therapy time a patient receives. Also, it reduces the risks of conflicting forms of patient management. There is an obvious disadvantage if a therapist is teaching a patient how to transfer from wheelchair to toilet, or hold a fork or spoon in one particular way, while the nursing staff, who may not be aware of these strategies, either train the patient differently or allow some other compensatory strategy to be displayed, thereby interfering with more appropriate skill acquisition.

Although the interdisciplinary method has proved a very successful and cost-effective way of providing therapy it seems difficult to introduce into the USA because the method of payment for rehabilitation is generally based on a fee-for-service, rather than *per diem* rate. It is ironic in this respect that the payment system for rehabilitation services in the USA is determining how treatment should be applied (and therefore what success can be achieved) rather than these factors being determined on the basis of good clinical judgement.

Generalization of training

The purpose of rehabilitation should be to provide the patient with skills that have 'life significance' and not just 'clinical significance'. For example, it is not sufficient to administer physical therapy with the aim of establishing independent mobility, if the treatment stops once the patient displays a reasonable gait pattern. Balance and endurance for walking should be assessed according to realistic criteria. Walking, as a form of behaviour, means walking somewhere! This may be to the local shopping precinct, into a bank, around a supermarket or onto a bus. Only when the patient can use walking skills independently in a community setting, can the goals of therapy be seen to be achieved.

The same criteria apply to all therapy. In speech therapy for example, the ability displayed by a patient to articulate speech clearly in the quiet of a therapy room does not constitute *talking*. Talking involves displaying speech skills under a variety of conditions, e.g. the noisy, pressured atmosphere of a supermarket, or some other setting where stress or some other important environmental factor may be present to interfere with the performance of that skill. As Hart and Hayden (1985) state:

> the ability to perform a task in a highly structured, quiet, one-to-one testing situation may not be at all reflective of [a patient's] ability to perform a similar task in a less structured, more distracting and informationally complex environment (p. 267).

Brown, Gordon and Diller (1985) make a similar point. They state that the tendency of assessment and remediation in rehabilitation has been to identify problems in the patient's daily life, evaluate the nature and extent of the deficit, then apply therapy and follow-up by a re-evaluation of the patient. Unfortunately, this process generally occurs 'within a milieu that may be quite different from that in which the 'service recipient' (the patient) must eventually implement the targeted skill.'

Evidence from experimental psychology should teach us that skills need to be practiced before they can be applied automatically, as a habit, with little conscious attention or disruption by external influences (Reason, 1984). We are rehabilitating behaviour, therefore the training process must offer the patient a chance to behave in as many situations as necessary in order for a skill to generalize and consolidate as a habit, because a habit has enduring properties which will not cease to operate once the patient has been discharged.

Evaluating and reporting

A considerable amount of effort has been applied to the development of scales or other devices to record progress and outcome in rehabilitation (see Chapter 12). In some respects the requirements vary according to the purpose of evaluation. If one is seeking to evaluate a whole system of rehabilitation then the measurement process is clearly going to be complex, diverse and quantitative. The requirements of an individual treatment programme are relatively straightforward, however, involving simple, single-case design methods, comparing changes that take place during treatment to a baseline measure of behaviour or ability that was recorded before treatment commenced. Examples of such methods are given in Wood (1978b) and a detailed explanation of methods and rationale is provided by Hersen and Barlow (1976).

The value of such approaches to treatment evaluation is that they can be used for the purpose of reporting progress in a clear and unambiguous way. Families, referring agencies, insurance personnel or independent case managers, find it easy to understand the rationale for further or different styles of treatment if they can actually see progress to a clearly defined goal (e.g. walking around a supermarket).

Too many reports in therapy are discipline orientated and convey information which is limited to one aspect of a patient's treatment. It is often difficult, after reading reports from all members of a treatment team, to condense the various activities and stated aims of therapy into a treatment plan which offers a clear understanding of the progress that has been achieved in respect of designated treatment goals. This can lead to confusion, misinterpretation of aims or results of treatment. More importantly, any misinterpretation of progress in relation to treatment goals might lead to treatment (or payment for treatment) being withdrawn prematurely.

SUMMARY

Rehabilitation is a process of teaching skills and abilities to individuals with physical and/or mental handicap. This implies a process of learning on the part of the patient, yet the apparatus which mediates learning, the brain, has been damaged and therefore, the learning mechanisms cannot be assumed to be operating efficiently! The salient factors approach to brain injury rehabilitation is an attempt to collect information about the nature of an individual's brain injury in order to understand how the learning system of a brain is operating. That knowledge is then applied to a rehabilitation treatment plan for the purpose of ameliorating the legacies of brain damage.

Implicit in this treatment model is the idea that the traditional framework of rehabilitation medicine is inadequate for the complex and diverse needs of 'brain function therapy' (Powell, 1981). Granger (1983) has suggested that the restricted utility of the medical model in rehabilitation is due, in part, to the differences which exist in a clinical setting designed to *care* for patients, as opposed to *curing* them. He feels that caring requires a different problem-solving approach, and while medicine is concerned with removing symptoms by identifying and removing the disease that produces the symptoms, the process of caring involves, in his words, 'a more burdensome and less heroic and more person-oriented level of managing the treatment of patients.'

Wood and Badley (1978) noted that the medical model is not suited to understanding disability and handicap because neither is exclusively a medical phenomenon and, indeed, the recent trend has been to emphasize social, cognitive and psychological factors as the essence of functional disability. As Granger (1983) stated:

> The challenge to the clinician is to understand the dynamics of the many varieties of functional limitations on a case by case basis and facilitate the management of the person with disability through a co-ordinated, long-term program (p. 21).

Coordinated, long-term rehabilitation programmes are not yet the norm, neither is the intradisciplinary approach upon which such concepts are based. In many ways, the maxim *tempora mutantur et nos mutamur inillis* (times change and we must change with them) is appropriate) to the development of brain injury rehabilitation at the moment. It will be of interest to monitor the diverse and complex changes that will need to occur in the existing (but not necessarily appropriate) treatment model over the next decade.

REFERENCES

Abrams, K.S., Neville, R. and Becker, M.C. (1973) Problem Oriented Recording of Psychosocial Problems. *Arch. Phys. Med. and Rehab.* **54**, 316–19.

Bond, M.R. (1984) The Psychiatry of Closed Head Injury, in *Closed Head Injury: Psychological, Social and Family Consequences* (D.N. Brooks, ed.), Oxford University Press, Oxford, pp. 148–78.

Bond, M.R. and Brooks, G.N. (1976) Understanding the Process of Recovery as a Basis for Rehabilitation of the Brain Injured. *Scand. J. Rehab. Med.*, **8**, 127–33.

Brooks, D.N. and McKinlay, W.W. (1983) Personality and Behavioural Change after Severe Blunt Head Injury. *J. Neurol., Neurosurg. Psychiat.*, **46**, 336–44.

Brown, M., Bordon, W.A. and Diller, L. (1985) Functional Assessment and Outcome Measurement: An Integrative Review, *Ann. Rev. Rehabil.*, **4**, 93–120.

Courville, C.B. (1945) *Pathology of the Nervous System*, 2nd edn, Pacific Press, California.

Diller, L., and Gordon, W.A. (1981) Criterion for Cognitive Deficit in Brain Injured Adults. *J. Consult. Clin. Psychol.*, **49**, 822–34.

Dresser, M., Meirowsky, A.M., Weiss, G.H. *et al.* (1973) Gainful Employment following Head Injury. *Arch. Neurol.*, **29**, 111–16.

Duckworth, D. (1983) The Need for a Standard Terminology and Classification of Disablement, in *Functional Assessment in Rehabilitation Medicine* (C.V. Granger and G.E. Gresham, eds), Williams and Wilkins, Baltimore.

Goldstein, G. (1983) Methodological and Theoretical Issues in Neuropsychological Assessment, in *Behavioural Assessment and Treatment of the Traumatically Brain Damaged* (R. Edelstein and E.C. Couture, eds), Plenum Press, New York.

Granger, C.V. (1983) A Conceptual Model for Functional Assessement, in *Functional Assessment in Rehabilitation Medicine* (C.V. Granger and G.E. Gresham, eds), Williams and Wilkins, Baltimore.

Groswasser, Z., Reider-Groswasser, M., Soroker, S. and Machtey, P. (1987) *Surg. Neurol.*, **27**, 331–37.

Hall, K. and Cope, N. (1985) The Current Status of Head Injury Rehabilitation, in *Neurotrauma. Treatment, Rehabilitation and Related Issues* (M.E. Millner and K. Wagner, eds), Butterworths, Boston.

Hart, T. and Hayden, M.E. (1985) The Current Status of Head Injury Rehabilitation, in *Neurotrauma. Treatment, Rehabilitation and Related Issues* (M.E. Millner and K. Wagner, eds), Butterworths, Boston.

Hersen, M. and Barlow, D.A. (1976) *Single Case Experimental Designs: Strategies for Studying Behaviour Change*, Pergamon, New York.

Jabbari, B., Venrow, M.I., Salazar, A.M. and Harper, M.G. (1986) Clinical and Radiological Correlates of EEG in the Late Phase of Head Injury; a Study of 515 Vietnam Veterans. *Electroencephalog. Clin. Neurophysio.*, **64**, 285–93.

Jamieson, K.J.G. and Kelly, D. (1973) Crash Helmets Reduce Head Injuries, *Med. J. Austr.*, **II**, 806.

Jennett, B. and Teasdale, G. (1981) *Management of Head Injuries*, F.A. Davies, Philadelphia.

Lezack, M.D. (1987) Assessment for Rehabilitation Planning, in *Neuropsychological Rehabilitation*. (M.J. Meier, A.L. Benton and L. Diller, eds), Churchill Livingstone, New York.

Lipper, M.A., Kishore, P.R.S., Enas, G.G. and Becker, D.P. (1985) Computer Tomography in the Prediction of Outcoming Head Injury. *J. Neuroradio.*, **6**, 7–10.

Mackworth, N.H. and Cope, D.N. (1982) *Towards an interpretation of Head Injury Recovery Trends*. The Head Injury Rehabilitation Project, Santa Clara Medical Center, San Jose. A report to the National Institute for Handicapped Research.

McQueen, J., Blackwood, D.H.R., Harris, P. *et al.* (1983) Low Risk of Late Post Traumatic Seizures following Severe Head Injury: Implications for Clinical Trials of Prophylaxis. *J. Neurol., Neurosurg. Psychiat.*, **46**, 899–904.

Newcombe, F. (1981) The Psychological Consequences of Closed Head Injury: Assessment and Rehabilitation. *Int. J. Rehabil. Med.*, **3**, 50–66.

Oddy, M.J., Humphrey, M.E. and Uttley, D. (1978) Subjectiave Impairment and Social Recovery after Closed Head Injury. *J. Neurol., Neurosurg. Psychiat.*, **41**, 611–16.

Posner, M. and Boies, S.J. (1971) Components of Attention. *Psycholog. Rev.*, **78**, 391–408.

Powell, G.E. (1981) *Brain Function Therapy*, Gower Publishing Company Limited, Aldershot, Hampshire.

Sarno, M.T. (1985) Functional Measurement in Verbal Impairment, Secondary to Brain Damage, in *Functional Assessment in Rehabilitation Medicine* (C.V. Granger and G.E. Gresham, eds), Williams and Wilkins, Baltimore.

Selgiman, M.E.T. (1975) *Helplessness: On Depression, Development and Death*, W.H. Freeman, San Francisco.

Stolov, W.C. (1982) Evaluation of the Patient, in *Handbook of Physical Medicine and Rehabilitation* (F.J. Kottke, G.K. Stillwell and J.F. Lehmann, eds), W.B. Sanders, Philadelphia.

Teuber, H.L. (1969) Neglected Aspects of the Post Traumatic Syndrome, in *The Late Effects of Head Injury* (A.E. Walker, W.F. Caveness and M. Critchley, eds), Charles C. Thomas, Springfield, Illinois.

Thomsen, I.V. (1984) Late Outcome of Very Severe Blunt Head Trauma: A 10/15 Year Second Follow-up. *J. Neurol., Neurosurg. Psychiat.*, **47**, 260–68.

Thompson, P.J. and Trimble, M.R. (1982) Anticonvulsant Drugs and Cognitive Function. *Epilepsia*, **23**, 531–44.

Walsh, K.W. (1978) *Neuropsychology: A Clinical Approach*, Churchill Livingstone, London and New York.

Willmore, W.F. (1985) Mechanisms and Management of Post Traumatic Epilepsy, in *Neutotrauma. Treatment, Rehabilitation and Related Issues* (M.E. Milner and K. Wagner, eds), Buttersworth, Boston.

Wood, P.H.N. and Badley, E.M. (1978) Setting Disablement in Perspective. *Int. Rehab. Med.*, **1**, 32–37.

Wood, R. Ll. (1987a) Neuropsychological Assessment in Brain Injury Rehabilitation, in *Advances in Rehabilitation* (M.G. Eisenbert and R.C. Grzesiak, eds), Springer Publishing Company, New York.

Wood, R. Ll. (1987b) *Brain Injury Rehabilitation: A Neurobehavioural Approach*, Croom Helm, London/Aspen Publishers, Rockville, MD.

7

The treatment of physical disorders following brain injury

Sheldon Berrol

The rehabilitation of physical problems resulting from traumatic brain injury represents a complex process that requires constant assessment of the patient's status, response to treatment, response to surgical and pharmacological interventions and of the process of spontaneous physiological recovery. The need for constant reassessment reflects the continual changes of these physical deficits through a variety of evolutionary stages. These changes demand awareness of a broad range of therapeutic approaches, appropriately timed, so as to maximize the results of ongoing intervention strategies (Berrol, 1985).

7.1 EARLY ACUTE INTERVENTIONS

An accurate diagnosis of residual physical problems must be documented as early as possible. Given their potential to change almost daily in the acute phase, the process of assessment must be incorporated into each treatment session.

Spasticity is a major motor problem during this and later stages. Since the patient may still be in coma, coordination and movement disorders can rarely be accurately determined. However, one can clearly determine the asymmetry of tone, reflex or synergy patterns that suggest the potential for manifest hemiplegia later.

The terms 'decorticate' and 'decerebrate' are commonly used to describe motor patterns in the comatose patient. The terms suggest an anatomical correlation with injury that in fact does not exist. It is far more useful for the neurosurgical and rehabilitation staff to describe the actual postures maintained at each joint. There appears to be prognostic significance to postures produced in response to stimulation (Jennett and Bond, 1975), and there may well be equal significance to static postures as well.

Sustained therapeutic interventions directed to the comatose patient with cerebral oedema can theoretically increase intracranial pressure. Postures such as bed flat, marked flexion of the hips and head rotation have been documented to do so (Durward *et al.*, 1983). The therapist should be well aware of this potential, and frequently observe the intracranial monitor for any consequences of such activities. Therapy sessions in the intensive care unit in general should be for shorter periods of time than usually designated for treatments on the ward.

7.2 RECOVERY FROM COMA

As the patient emerges from coma, there is frequently a change from extensor to flexor pattern of the upper extremities, while the extensor pattern of the lower extremities is maintained. Plantar flexion becomes predominant in the ankle. This shift in tone with its resultant postures generally heralds the return of intrinsic automatic control. It is at this time that various automatisms of motor function begin. Painful stimuli may induce a strong flexor pattern of the lower extremities. If this persists, ambulation may be interfered with at a later stage. It is important therefore, to avoid repeated nocioceptive stimuli that may habituate such motor responses and induce abnormal patterns (Boughton and Ciesla, 1986).

The process of recovery can be facilitated by an awareness of potential effects, positive or negative, of routine nursing procedures. For example, in an attempt to prevent plantar flexion contractures of the ankle, foot-boards may sometimes be used in bed. The positional pressure provided by foot-boards is generally over the heads of the metatarsals, thus facilitating the spastic reflex of the ankle plantar flexors. While such devices may prevent 'windswept' (varus-valgus) deformities of the feet, they also facilitate an increase in spasticity with its resultant potential for contractures.

Range of motion

Range of motion exercises should be performed not only by the therapy staff, but as part of routine nursing treatment (such as bed baths, patient turning etc.). This requires that nursing staff become intimately involved as part of the rehabilitation team, even in the intensive care unit. Such full range of motion should be administered at least once each shift (three times a day). The range of motion provided should be maximal, performed with slow but steady passive stretch, and the maximal range maintained for several seconds before release. Families should be carefully instructed in such procedures, so that the frequency of exercise is increased. They should also be instructed and supervised in providing tactile stimulation appropriately. If the patient is obviously hemiplegic, family members should direct their efforts to the less involved side. It must be noted that in spite of the most aggressive application of range of motion exercises, contractures may ensue (Perry, 1983; Carr and Shepherd, 1980).

Sensory stimulation

Interventions should provide appropriately directed sensory stimuli (Griffin, 1974). Overly aggressive stimuli may induce generalized startle reactions, bruxism, chewing reflexes etc., that result in a habituated pattern that may be difficult to modify later. The programme should be carefully planned and monitored with a goal of obtaining as normal a response as possible. Stimuli should be introduced singly and for short periods of time; each should be novel enough to induce a response, but not of such intensity that defensive motoric reactions are obtained. At present, there is little evidence of the therapeutic value of such programmes, but the monitoring of response that it requires certainly allows for earlier recognition of meaningful responses than more conventional methods of assessment.

As automatic motor behaviours evolve, they should be identified and incorporated into the treatment programme. In general, one should be careful not to continue to facilitate abnormal reflex patterns that could potentially interfere with later functional movement (Rood, 1962). Occasionally, reflexes such as the asymmetric tonic neck reflex may be induced to facilitate functional activities such as reaching.

7.3 SPASTICITY

Management of spasticity requires a holistic perspective throughout the many phases of recovery. It is generally the most pervasive long-term motor problem that must be dealt with. It is manifested by an exaggerated stretch reflex that produces an increase in resistance to passive stretch that is rate dependent, a pattern of hyper-reflexia exemplified by increased deep tendon reflexes, clonus and the clasped knife phenomena. The increase in tonus is generally asymmetrical, thus contributing to the major complication, contracture. As muscle shortens through the process of contracture, the gamma bias becomes reset, increasing the frequency and level of spasticity. Thus a primary objective in early management is to maintain the normal length of muscle fibres (Perry, 1983; Glenn and Rosenthal, 1985).

The initial approach to managing spasticity is the avoidance of any cutaneous nocioceptive factor that may facilitate increases in tone and prolonged shortening of muscle. Factors responsible for initiating such a response include anything that may induce pain. Thus prompt attention to any skin breakdown, bladder distension, ingrown toenails etc., may reduce the overall level of spasticity, simplifying management.

Positioning

The severely head-injured patient assumes prolonged postures that facilitate the development of spasticity and contractures. Maintenance of these postures produces structural change in muscle tissue and muscle spindle morphology and alteration of muscle spindle receptivity (Ashby, 1976). Proper patient positioning in bed and wheelchair can inhibit this tendency. Appropriate positioning allows us to achieve more complete range of motion in a static position, and facilitates normal movement patterns. Reflex-inhibiting patterns should be utilized as frequently as possible (for example, avoiding pressure over the metatarsal heads by using large foot-plates in the wheelchair). Segmental control should be established both distally and proximally (Shaw, 1986).

The upright position can accelerate a decrease in tone, and provide for increased kinesthetic, tactile, visual and vestibular input. Oral feeding, alerting and body awareness are facilitated.

Tone in the hand, wrist and finger flexors can be reduced by abduction and external rotation of the thumb. This posture should therefore be adopted prior to application of orthotic devices, and incorporated into orthotic design (Snook, 1979). In developing functional hand activities of a volitional nature in the presence of spasticity, this procedure should be part of routine 'warm up'. Maintaining the shoulder at 90 degrees of abduction will similarly reduce the tone in the upper extremity, and this position should be encouraged for specific time intervals during the day, whenever the patient is in bed.

Flexion of the hips and knees to slightly greater than 90 degrees will inhibit generalized extensor tone, making it desirable to incorporate this posture into the general nursing plan as well as into wheelchair design. Side-lying in itself is inhibitory, and in this position, the knee-flexed posture can frequently be easily integrated. The knee-hip flexed posture should be integrated with a rigid wheelchair seat to prevent the tendency towards adduction contracture promoted by sling seats. The use of lap boards and/or restraining hip bars can also assist in maintaining the proper degree of flexion at the hips. Additional stabilizing devices to properly align the patient may include lateral trunk supports, chest straps, suspender restraints, head control supports and adductor wedges.

Appropriate wheelchair positioning can be a useful therapeutic modality in the management of spasticity (Motloch, 1977; Shaw, 1986). The sitting devices frequently used in acute and intensive care settings, such as 'cardiac chairs' should be avoided since they promote increased tone and subsequent deformity.

Head positioning

Maintaining proper head posture in the wheelchair is frequently a most difficult problem. A restraining device is commonly necessary, and since each case is so unique individual manufacture of each device is usually essential. In general, such devices should avoid prolonged pressure over the mandibular condyle. Straps that encompass the chin and direct pressure upwards may add to existing temporomandibular joint problems that first become manifest when the patient later becomes more aware. Commercially available head restraint systems have a limited ability to conform to individual problems, and at times may contribute to discomfort, pressure problems etc.

A word of caution regarding those abnormal head positions that represent a compensation for extra-occular muscle dysfunction. While the general tendency is to align the head vertically, in the presence of cranial nerve IV (superior oblique muscle) paresis, patients frequently assume a head-tilt that permits adequate alignment of the horizon. Since this muscle is a primary intorter of the eye, loss of this function requires head-tilting for compensation.

A head-turned position should alert one to evaluate the potential for other visual system problems before developing alignment devices. These include visual field loss and nystagmus.

7.4 MODALITIES

The primary approach to spasticity management is the stretching of muscle fibre to maintain its normal length. This principle is basic in the use of casting and splinting techniques. These procedures additionally reduce cutaneous receptor stimulation. Once a maximal range of motion has been obtained (even if only temporarily), then encouragement of isolated movement is incorporated into the treatment plan. A variety of physical modalities have a role in the treatment process.

Splints and serial casts

Prevention of muscle shortening should be a primary goal in the intensive care unit. This generally requires the use of resting splints and/or
casts to maintain functional ranges of motion. Prefabricated ankle-foot
orthoses generally do not conform to tissue adequately, and may
therefore produce abrasions and ultimately tissue breakdown in the
presence of spasticity (Cusick and Sussman, 1982). In addition, such
devices do not provide the circumferential tissue pressure necessary to
reduce cutaneous receptor stimulation. Casts, by their very nature, do
meet both of these requirements. If the range of motion has been
reduced substantially, then serial application of casts may be called for.
The use of drop-out casts may permit access by the therapist to joints
that continue to need dynamic stretching. Casts may be bivalved
when adequate range of motion has been achieved, so that the
extremity can be adequately evaluated and treated during the therapy
session. There is evidence, however, that the non-bivalved cast may be
more effective in maintaining the range of motion, and may be
associated with a lower incidence of skin breakdown. High-topped
shoes rarely prove therapeutic, and will obscure a developing foot
drop. Additionally, they may increase the level of spasticity since
failure to adequately immobilize the joint may actually increase the
tone through stimulation of cutaneous receptors (Gans *et al.*, 1979).

Upper extremity splinting or casts may be indicated when flexor
tone is increased, or when spasticity results in shortening of elbow,
wrist and/or finger flexors. Again the value of circumferential pressure
may dictate the use of casts rather than splints to maintain the
position. In the early stages of management, maintenance of position
of function may be adequate; as spasticity progresses, however, devices
that provide for maximal extension should be introduced as rapidly as
tolerated to stretch the muscle groups at greatest risk for contracture,
the flexors (Snook, 1979). The wrist should be maintained in a
position of extension, and then metacarpophalangeal and inter-
phalangeal joints in extension or at least neutral.

Serial casting is an effective therapeutic approach in the presence of
developing or developed contractures. The maintenance of an
increased range of motion by plaster application, reintroduction of
dynamic stretch with reapplication of plaster in a serial fashion, has
substantially reduced the number of surgical muscle-lengthening
procedures in this patient population (Keenan, 1987). The use of nerve
blocks or motor point blocks prior to cast application may dramatically
reduce the number of cast applications required. Casts must conform
well enough to skin so as to avoid friction effect, incorporate sufficient

padding over bony prominences to prevent pressure injury and be loose enough to prevent any constriction that could produce oedema. The use of these techniques dictates the need for frequent evaluation of the limb, and caution in the presence of sensory loss, peripheral vascular impairment, diabetes etc.

Heat

Thermal modalities can induce local and general relaxation that may allow greater stretch of muscle. Increased local temperature can increase the 'creeping action' of viscoelastic tissue and induce reflex inhibition of spastic muscle (Lehmann *et al.*, 1970; Lehmann and DeLateur, 1982a). There is little if any advantage of heating machines over local hot packs or the therapeutic pool. In addition, heated therapeutic pools may facilitate volitional muscle activity through the inherent buoyancy of water. It can also be used as a prelude relaxing modality prior to 'dry' exercise programmes. The patient must be evaluated, however, for any negative effect on endurance that may be produced.

Cold

Cryotherapy has long been used to reduce localized spasticity prior to range of motion exercises (Eldrede *et al.*, 1960). Cutaneously applied ice inhibits gamma spasticity by reducing the discharge rate of the muscle spindle afferents, when applied for approximately 10 minutes. The duration of action is quite short (20 minutes), and thus its greatest utility is in the therapy treatment session. Empirically, it appears to have the additional advantage of pain relief (Lehmann and Delateur, 1982b). When used to stimulate stretch receptors, Rood (1962) stresses that brisk icing must be applied over the dermatomes whose nerve supply coincides with the muscle to be stimulated.

Vibration

At low frequencies, vibration over agonist muscles can suppress hyper-reflexia. Higher frequency vibration may be applied to antagonist muscles, thereby facilitating contraction and concomitant inhibition of spastic muscles. This may be quite helpful in re-education of extremely paretic muscle. If, however, vibration is applied directly over spastic muscle, it can enhance the tone not only in the involved muscle, but in those muscles that contribute to the synergy pattern of the limb as well (Hagbarth and Ecklund, 1966; 1968).

Ultrasound

Ultrasound exerts its primary effect through heat produced at tissue interfaces. As with other heating modalities, it increases the extensibility of soft tissue by altering the intrinsic viscoelastic state towards more fluidity, allowing greater length of muscle fibre to be obtained. It may therefore be of value prior to a dynamic stretching intervention. Of additional value is the decrease in reflex muscle spindle excitability that it causes.

Electrical stimulation

At present, electrical stimulation has little application in the acute phase of management. When the patient develops sufficient attentional capacity and can actively participate, this modality can be quite useful in motor re-education, providing auditory and/or visual feedback for motor control. Functional electrical stimulation (FES) can not only trigger contraction of individual muscles, but of those muscles involved in patterns of movement. In addition, FES suppresses the antagonist spastic muscle contractions (demonstrating Sherrington's Law of Reciprocal Innervation). This technique may have some long-term motor learning effect as well (Baker *et al.*, 1983; Zablotney, 1987).

7.5 DRUG THERAPY

When physical approaches alone fail to accomplish adequate results in reducing spasticity to functional levels, then pharmacological interventions may be considered. It is important to recognize, however, that medication to reduce spasticity will not affect an established contracture. The presence of fixed contracture at one or more major joints should also raise the question of underlying heterotopic ossification (see below).

As long as the patient demonstrates motor improvement, spasticity need not be treated with medication. When there is obvious failure to progress, then additional interventions may become necessary. If the spasticity produces pain, then it should be treated since any nociceptive cutaneous, myopathic or somatic input may increase overall tonus.

Any agent that sedates the patient may decrease the level of spasticity. In dealing with a patient who already has problems of alerting, arousal and attention however, such drug interventions should be used with caution. Currently three pharmacological interventions are available that have demonstrated a primary effect upon upper motor neuron (UMN) spasticity. (Drugs that are designed for 'muscle spasm' of a peripheral origin are primarily sedative and have no role in the management of UMN spasticity.)

1. Diazepam acts suprasegmentally in depressing motor tone, but produces inhibition at the internuncial neuronal pool at the spinal level as well. However, it is a well documented sedative (with associated cognitive depressant effect), and because of specific diazepam receptor sites within brain tissue, it is habituating. Since it is also an analeptic agent, sudden discontinuance may lead to seizure.

2. Dantrolene sodium acts peripherally in muscle tissue, controlling the release of calcium from the sarcoplasmic reticulum. It thus produces an initial generalized weakness that abates in some 5 to 7 days. (For a patient in the agitated phase, this may be of some value.) It is, however, potentially hepatotoxic, and thus liver function studies should be performed prior to initiating therapy and reassessed routinely during administration. Dantrolene sodium appears to be more effective in cerebrally-induced, than spinally-induced spasticity.

3. Baclofen appears to act centrally at the spinal internuncial cell pool. As a result, it is more effective in spinally-induced spasticity. There appears to be some suprasegmental effect as well, since confusion, agitation and/or hallucination may occur in some patients.

Combinations of these drugs may be synergistic in cases where single drug management is ineffective. The goal of therapy is not to eliminate spasticity, but to modulate it, to reduce the power of the spastic muscle. Drugs should be used as an adjuvant, not as a substitute for a programme of physical restoration (Glenn and Rosenthal, 1985).

Neurolytic blocks

Severely head-injured patients often require additional procedures. Anaesthetic agents for local blocks can be used with great advantage in distinguishing fixed contracture from spasticity, or in an attempt to gain greater range of motion prior to application of serial casts (Keenan, 1987).

Neurolytic agents such as phenol or alcohol can produce longer-lasting effects. Occasionally alcohol washes have been used to infiltrate the muscle mass, but this non-specific approach requires larger quantities of medication, frequent re-injection and may contribute to more extensive fibrosis within tissue (Carpenter and Seitz, 1980).

Motor point block or nerve blocks are preferable, since greater precision can be accomplished (Petrillo et al., 1980). Percutaneous blocks are performed with a teflon-coated needle, whose tip also functions as a muscle or nerve stimulator, allowing minimal medication. Phenol 3-6% is the most frequently administered medication. Blocks of nerves which have both motor and sensory components are best performed under open surgical procedure (Khalili et al., 1964).

Although such procedures are most commonly introduced later in the rehabilitation process when specific functional goals can be identified, they are very useful early on in localized problems. One such early indication is the severely flexed non-functional elbow with severe spasticity. Percutaneous or open phenol block of the musculocutaneous nerve can obviate later need for tendon-lengthening procedures (Braun et al., 1973; Garland, Blum and Waters, 1980).

7.6 SURGERY

Surgical interventions for spasticity in severe head injury are designed to lengthen or release muscle. Surgery may therefore be thought of as an extension of stretching techniques (Keenan, 1987).

The most frequently performed intervention is the lengthening of the Achilles' tendon. Unfortunately, this procedure alone may leave the foot and ankle with motor imbalance, resulting in greater deformity. Prior to any such surgical intervention, a comprehensive evaluation of the motor system is essential, determining the level of spasticity in agonist and antagonist muscles. Polyelectromyographic evaluation may contribute substantially to an understanding of the imposing forces and identify the extent of surgery necessary to produce a balanced extremity (Keenan et al., 1984). In selected cases of drop foot with equinovarus position, tendon transfer such as the split anterior tibialis transfer combined with lengthening of the Achilles' tendon and release of toe flexors may maximize function, reduce spasticity and eliminate the need for bracing (Rush, 1983).

The decision to intervene surgically must result from a team analysis. Although the choice of surgical technique is solely within the province of the orthopaedic surgeon, the indications for intervention, timing of such intervention, and planning for the pre- and post-operative phases rests with the entire therapeutic team.

For those patients who demonstrate little to no improvement over the course of their rehabilitation phase, and whose level of spasticity interferes with routine nursing care and positioning or produces significant pain, percutaneous radiofrequency rhizotomy may offer substantial benefit in selected cases (Kasdon and Lathia, 1984). There is rarely an indication for more radical procedures such as chordotomy or myelotomy in brain-injured survivors.

7.7 HETEROTOPIC OSSIFICATION

Heterotopic ossification (HO) occurs commonly in patients with severe head injuries. The frequency appears to increase with increasing extent of brain tissue loss and length of coma (Sazbon et al., 1981). Three factors may be responsible for initiation of the process, a traumatic, a neurogenic and/or a vascular aspect. Most frequent sites are the hip, shoulders and elbows in head injury (Garland, Blum and Waters, 1980).

Aetiology

Local trauma to long bone may result in an excessive proliferation of callus formation, leading in its extreme, to ankylosis of a joint. Additionally, in central nervous system trauma, the presence of healing bone may lead to calcification and ossification of a joint or joints peripheral to the trauma.

A neurogenic factor has been suspected but is as yet unidentified. Ossification about joints not exposed to local trauma occurs with significant frequency; although the older literature suggested that this is a result of aggressive mobilization of the involved joint, no substantive evidence of this thesis has yet been presented.

Early triple phase bone scan evaluation of joints that eventually develop HO characteristically demonstrate increased local blood flow. It is reasonable to presume therefore, that there is a vascular component in the development of HO.

Diagnosis

The initial phase of HO development is usually associated with the onset of local swelling, erythema, increased local temperature and decreased range of motion. It is thus clinically compatible with an acute thrombophlebitis. A differential diagnosis must be established rapidly, since the treatment approach for each is so different.

There is a characteristic increase in alkaline phosphatase concentrations when new bone is being formed. Such elevations are present when a fracture is healing, when growth is occurring (children and teenagers), and in a variety of liver conditions. The elevation of alkaline phosphatase in HO begins after the calcification process has begun. X-ray findings at this stage may be negative. Bone scan studies can identify the process quite early, before alkaline phosphatase and X-ray studies become positive.

The evaluation that most often leads to the diagnosis is serial range of motion testing. Lack of progress in the daily range of motion programme (especially if there is no change in the level of spasticity) should lead one to suspect the possibility of underlying ossifying tissue. Daily measurements of each extremity will contribute further information regarding the development of concomitant oedema.

Treatment

Drug therapy

Ossification and thus ankylosis may be prevented or decreased through the early use of disodium etidronate (Spielman et al., 1984). It is frequently difficult, however, to identify the patient who is predisposed to the development of HO and the drug cannot reverse abnormal bone formation.

Physical modalities such as ultrasound and diathermy appear not to be of benefit. Theoretically, early use of these techniques may be deleterious by their local effect of increased vascular flow.

Passive range of motion is the mainstay of management in developing HO. The development of a pseudoarthrosis in ossifying tissue may preserve substantial function. The potential for microtrauma as a precipitating factor, while a real potential, appears to have been overstated in the past. Extremities should be positioned at all times to maintain range, and therefore preserve function. Splints should be utilized for limited periods of time in joints at risk. Spasticity should be controlled as well as possible, since it may contribute to increasing levels of HO. The same has been reported with the presence of decubiti.

Surgery

Surgical removal of the ossification that has ankylosed a joint may be considered at approximately 18 months post-injury, when maximal motor recovery will have been attained. The most satisfactory results are obtained in the patients with reasonable motor control of the involved extremity. Ideally, patients should be premedicated with disodium etidronate and maintained for 3 months post-surgery.

Manipulation of HO under anaesthesia appears to be a promising alternative to surgical intervention in selected cases (Garland et al., 1982).

7.8 ATAXIA

Disorders of coordination commonly occur after traumatic brain injury. Cerebellar ataxia can severely limit the re-learning of functional skills, and represent one of the most difficult sequelae of motor dysfunction. Although spasticity and motor weakness can occasionally present as tremor, dysmetria and incoordination, true deficits of coordination become clearly identified by serial evaluations.

Ataxia results in inaccurate, but not inappropriate, motor control. It may result from damage to the cerebellum, subcortical structures or the brain-stem, and recovery proceeds at a slow, at times imperceptible rate. The rehabilitation of ataxia requires the recalibration of motor performance. To obtain this, there is a need for continual feedback in the treatment process, using auditory, tactile and visual feedback systems. The feedback must be immediate to promote accurate information acquisition, and there is a critical need for repetition. Deterioration in the rate of motor learning in the presence of fatigue is greater than with spasticity (Brudny et al., 1977).

Tasks must be introduced in an hierarchical fashion, gradually adding to the complexity. The involved extremity should be evaluated to determine the least stable joint, and then joint stability provided. This can at times be accomplished by weighting, or bracing that allows a single, previously determined plane of movement. Bracing is, however, rarely tolerated for very long and so should be used mainly for the initiation of functional activity.

Weighting can be applied to virtually any limb joint, or to an adaptive device such as splint, shoe, spoon, walker or even vests for truncal stability. The added stimulus to proprioceptive receptors acts as its own potent biofeedback device. Strengthening selected muscle groups may also increase stability and functional ability (Carr and Shepherd, 1980).

In those patients who are so disabled by ataxia that basic activities of daily living cannot be accomplished, in spite of substantial cognitive gains, stereotaxic thalamotomy may be considered. Results of this procedure in appropriate cases appear promising (Andrew, 1981; Andrew et al., 1982; Bullard and Nashold, 1984).

7.9 MOBILIZATION

Mobilization is in itself a stretching activity, as well as an intense sensory and proprioceptive input activity. The process is impeded in the presence of contractures and may be facilitated by orthotic devices designed to combat contractures and spasticity. The use of the upright position achieved by wheelchair or standing frame provides more intensive stimulation than can be achieved by a bed-bound programme of therapy.

Tilt tables may be used initially to adapt the cardiovascular system to the upright position. If postural hypertension occurs, then abdominal binders and/or elastic wraps of the lower extremities can help to stabilize blood pressure. The patient should be advanced to a standing frame as rapidly as possible since it provides more proprioceptive and vestibular stimulation as well as greater stretch on the heel cords and hip musculature. This gravity-assisted sustained stretching is more effective than manually provided stretching. The standing frame also allows for multiple stimulation techniques to be provided simultaneously. Mirrors can add the dimension of visual feedback for motor activities. Joint approximation can also be provided more effectively in the upright position. It is not uncommon for patients to feed more effectively in this position than in bed or seated.

Mats or plinths facilitate therapeutic exercises, and overcome the limitations imposed by a hospital bed. They should be at least double sized to allow full body rotation. In general, the training of functional activities should proceed in a developmental sequence. Since each aspect of the sequence facilitates subsequent performance requirements, it employs a 'building block' approach to motor activities (Carr and Shepherd, 1980).

7.10 VOLITIONAL CONTROL

Motor control develops in several stages. It is essential that the task requirements fall within the capability of the individual. This requires the therapist to perform task analysis in an hierarchical fashion for each anticipated goal. After mobilization has been adequately established, concentration on stability of both segments and the whole (maintenance of postures) are required prior to controlled mobility activities. The final phase of motoric reintegration focuses on skill development.

Patients should not be advanced to ambulation activities until they are able to follow basic instructions to transfer safely, can stabilize the hips and knees, have volitional control of hip musculature and have tolerable limits of contractures of the lower extremities. Initiation of ambulation training requires two therapists so that adequate provision of stabilization, feedback, cueing and safety can be provided.

Occasionally specific neurological treatment approaches are

developed that require adherence to a doctrinaire philosophy. This demands that brain injury be perceived as a homogeneous diagnostic category. It is, however, widely recognized that different patterns of injury exist within the brain-injured population and that they therefore require individual management approaches. Recent studies suggest that a broader view of therapeutic intervention strategies is of substantial patient benefit.

7.11 SUMMARY

Physical management of the severely brain-injured patient is a long and protracted process. Time limitations on this may exist, but are not uncommonly a result of knowledge limitations of individual clinicians. Proper management dictates that the process begins in the intensive care unit. The patients' problems change over time, and so must the rehabilitation process if effect is to be maximized. Constant reassessment is essential, so that the goals set for the patient can become more realistic over time. Specific rehabilitation approaches must be designed to anticipate problems, and to intervene appropriately as these changes occur.

The rehabilitation therapist should identify those pre-morbid motor activities that can be learned, and which must be compensated for. Even when decisions are made to compensate for a specific function, sufficient change may occur over time that leads to a potential for greater motor learning, which then requires changes in intervention strategies. Rehabilitation must encompass achievable short-term goals as well as long-term goals. Paramount amongst the goals is the prevention of complications.

Finally, one most recognize that improved motor ability allows greater control over the environment and facilitates the process of cognitive reintegration.

REFERENCES

Andrew, J. (1981) Surgery for Involuntary Movements. *Br. J. Hosp. Med.*, **26**, 522–28.

Andrew, J., Fowler, C.J. and Harrison, M.J.G. (1982) Tremor After Head Injury and Its Treatment by Stereotactic Surgery. *J. Neurol., Neurosurg. Psychiat.*, **45**, 815–19.

Ashby, P. (1976) Neurophysiologic Changes in Hemiplegia: Possible Explanation for the Disparity Between Muscle Tone and Tendon Reflexes. *Neurology*, **26**, 1145–51.

Baker, L.L., Parker, K. and Sanderson, D. (1983) Neuromuscular Electrical

Stimulation for the Head Injured Patient. *Phys. Ther.*, **63**, 1967–74.

Berrol, S. (1985) The Rehabilitation Process. *Seminars in Neurol.*, **5**, 205–11.

Boughton, A. and Ciesla, N. (1986) Physical Therapy Management of the Head-Injured Patient in the Intensive Care Unit. *Topics in Acute Care Trauma Rehabil.*, **1**, 1–18.

Braun, R.M., Hoffer, M.M. and Mooney, V. (1973) Phenol Nerve Block in the Treatment of Acquired Spastic Hemiplegia in the Upper Limb. *J. Bone Joint Surg.*, **55-A**, 580–85.

Brudny, J., Korein, J. and Grynbaum, B.B. (1977) Sensory Feedback Therapy in Patients with Brain Insult. *Scand. J. Rehabil. Med.*, **9**, 155–63.

Bullard, D.E. and Nashold, B.S. (1984) Stereotaxic Thalamotomy for the Treatment of Posttraumatic Movement Disorders. *J. Neurosurg.*, **61**, 316–21.

Carpenter, E.B. and Seitz, D.G. (1980) Intramuscular Alcohol as an Aid in the Management of Spastic Cerebral Palsy. *Dev. Med. Child. Neurol.*, **22**, 497–501.

Carr, J.H. and Shepherd, R.B. (eds) (1980) *A Clinical Guide. Physiotherapy in Disorders of the Brain*, Heinemann, London.

Cusick, B.C. and Sussman, M.D. (1982) Short Leg Casts: Their Role in Management of Cerebral Palsy. *Phys. Occ. Ther. Ped.*, **2**, 93–95.

Durward, Q.J., Amacher, A.L., Del Maestro, R.F. and Sibbald, W.J. (1983) Cerebral and Cardiovascular Responses to Changes in Head Elevation in Patients with Intracranial Hypertension. *J. Neurosurg.*, **59**, 938–44.

Eldrede, S., Lindsley, D.F. and Buchwald, J.S. (1960) The Effect of Cooling on Mammalian Muscle Spindles. *Exp. Neurol.*, **2**, 144–57.

Gans, B.M., Erickson, G. and Simons, D. (1979) Below-Knee Orthosis: A Wrap-Around Design for Ankle-Foot Control. *Arch. Phys. Med. Rehabil.*, **60**, 78–80.

Garland, D.E., Blum, C. and Waters, R.L. (1980) Pariarticular Heterotopic Ossification in Head Injured Adults. Incidence and Location. *J. Bone Joint Surg.*, **62-A**, 942–46.

Garland, D.E., Thompson, R. and Waters, R.L. (1980) Musculocutaneous Neurectomy for Spastic Elbow Flexion in Non-Functional Upper Extremities in Adults. *J. Bone Joint Surg.*, **62-A**, 108–12.

Garland, D.E., Razza, B. and Waters, R.L. (1982) Forceful Joint Manipulation in Head Injured Adults with Heterotopic Ossification. *Clin. Ortho.*, **169**, 133–38.

Glenn, M.B. and Rosenthal, M. (1985) Rehabilitation Following Severe Traumatic Brain Injury. *Seminars in Neurol.*, **5**, 233–46.

Griffin, J.W. (1974) Use of Proprioceptive Stimuli in Therapeutic Exercise. *Phys. Ther.*, **54**, 1072–79.

Hagbarth, K.E. and Eklund, G. (1966) Tonic Vibration Reflexes (TVR) in Spasticity. *Brain Res.*, **2**, 201–3.

Hagbarth, K.E. and Ecklund, G. (1968) The Effect of Muscle Vibration in Spasticity, Rigidity and Cerebellar Disorders. *J. Neurol. Neurosurg. Psychiat.*, **31**, 207–13.

Jennett, B. and Bond, M. (1975) Assessment of Outcome after Severe Brain Damage. *Lancet*, **i**, 480.

Kasdon, D.L. and Lathia, E.S. (1984) A Prospective Study of Radiofrequency Rhizotomy in the Treatment of Posttraumatic Spasticity. *Neurosurg.*, **15**, 526–29.

Keenan, M.A.E. (1987) The Orthopedic Management of Spasticity. *J. Head Trauma Rehabil.*, **2**, 57–61.

Keenan, M., Creighton, J. and Garland, D.E. (1984) Surgical Correction of Spastic Equinovarus Deformity in the Adult Head Trauma Patient. *Foot and Ankle*, **5**, 35–41.

Khalili, A.A., Harmel, M.H. and Forster, S. (1964) Management of Spasticity by Selective Peripheral Nerve Block with Dilute Phenol Solutions in Clinical Rehabilitation. *Arch. Phys. Med. Rehabil.*, **45**, 513–19.

Lehmann, J.F. and DeLateur, B.J. (1982a) Therapeutic Heat, in *Therapeutic Heat and Cold*, J.F. Lehmann (ed.), Williams and Wilkins, Baltimore, pp. 404–562.

Lehmann, J.F. and DeLateur, B.J. (1982b) Cryotherapy, in *Therapeutic Heat and Cold*, J.F. Lehmann (ed.), Williams and Wilkins, Baltimore, pp. 563–602.

Lehmann, J.F., Masock, A.J. and Warren, C.G. (1970) Effect of Therapeutic Temperatures on Tendon Extensibility. *Arch. Phys. Med. Rehabil.*, **51**, 481–87.

Motloch, W.M. (1977) Seating and Posturing for the Physically Impaired. *Orthotics Prosthetics*, **31**, 11–21.

Perry, J. (1983) Rehabilitation of the Neurologically Disabled Patient: Principles, Practice, and Scientific Basis. *J. Neurosurg.*, **58**, 799–816.

Petrillo, C.R., Chu, D.S. and Davis, S.W. (1980) Phenol Block of the Tibial Nerve in the Hemiplegic Patient. *Orthopedics*, **3**, 871–74.

Rood, M. (1962) The Use of Sensory Receptors to Activate and Inhibit Motor Response, Autonomic and Somatic in Developmental Sequence, in *Approaches to Treatment of Patients with Neuromuscular Dysfunction*, C. Sattely (ed.), Brown & Co., Dubuque.

Rush, G.A. (1983) Split Anterior Tibial Tendon Transfer, *Contemp. Ortho.*, **7**, 51–57.

Sazbon, L., Najenson, T. and Tartakovsky, M.M. (1981) Widespread Periarticular New-Bone Formation in Long-Term Comatose Patients. *J. Bone Joint Surg.*, **63**, 120–25.

Shaw, R. (1986) Persistent Vegetative State: Principles and Techniques for Seating and Positioning. *J. Head Trauma Rehabil.*, **1**, 31–37.

Snook, J.H. (1979) Spasticity Reduction Splint. *Am. J. Occ. Ther.*, **33**, 648–51.

Spielman, G., Gennareli, T. and Rogers, R.C. (1984) Disodium Etidronate: Its Role in Preventing Heterotopic Ossification in Severe Head Injury. *Arch. Phys. Med. Rehabil.*, **64**, 539–42.

Zablotny, C. (1987) Using Neuromuscular Electrical Stimulation to Facilitate Limb Control in the Head-Injured Patient. *J. Head Trauma Rehabil.*, **2**, 28–33.

8 Models of cognitive rehabilitation

Barbara Wilson

If we take cognition to refer to processes involved in knowing, understanding, learning, perceiving, attending, remembering and judging, then a cognitive deficit is an impairment to one or more of these processes, resulting in a loss of efficiency or reduction of function.

Cognitive rehabilitation attempts to remediate, ameliorate or alleviate cognitive deficits that have resulted from brain injury. The term 'cognitive rehabilitation' can apply to any intervention strategy or technique which intends to enable clients or patients and their families to live with, manage, bypass, reduce or come to terms with cognitive deficits precipitated by injury to the brain.

It is an essential requirement that a cognitive rehabilitation programme is properly monitored and evaluated in order to estimate its contribution towards improvement in one or more of the affected processes. Without proper monitoring and evaluation we can never be sure whether improvement has simply resulted from natural recovery or some other non-specific factor unrelated to treatment. Programmes that are not properly evaluated cannot inform the design of future programmes. Those that are evaluated properly will encourage better designs and the development of a sturdier theoretical framework within which to work in the future.

A severe head injury can cause deficits that are not cognitive. For example, it can cause problems that can be defined as motor, sensory, behavioural, emotional, or as disturbances of the personality. It is necessary, therefore, when selecting the goals and treatment techniques for cognitive rehabilitation, to be aware not only of the number and range of problems to be confronted, but also to ascertain whether those problems are indeed cognitive by nature. If we consider, for example, patients who, having suffered some kind of injury to the brain, exhibit symptoms of anxiety and fearfulness, then we need to know whether these symptoms are emotional, cognitive or behavioural manifestations of the injury. These questions are illustrated in Table 8.1, which contains diagnoses of three patients who were referred for

Table 8.1 Diagnosis of patients with fear and anxiety problems

Description of problem	Cause of brain damage	Classification of problem
Fear of hydrotherapy pool. Always been frightened of water	Right cerebrovascular accident	Emotional problem? Independent of brain damage.
Fear of physiotherapy due to contractures, pain and previous inappropriate treatment	Severe head injury	Behaviour problem? Exhibited after brain damage. Indirect result of brain damage.
Fear of walking alone and of transferring	Right cerebrovascular accident	Cognitive problem? Loss of depth and distance perception. Direct result of brain damage

help with problems involving fear and anxiety.

Apraxia is another condition which is not always easy to classify. It is a disorder of movement but it cannot be explained in terms of weakness, paralysis or poor comprehension. Unlike some other disorders of movement, it cannot be classified solely as a motor problem because it does not result from weaknesses to the motor system but rather to planning or voluntary control of the motor processes; and in this sense it can be regarded as a cognitive problem. However, a more accurate description would have to admit that it appears to be a problem that crosses the boundaries of both motor and cognitive deficits.

Even when it is clear that a problem is cognitive by nature and source we may experience difficulty in placing it within its specific category or type of cognitive problem. Take, for example, the case of a patient with a good motor ability who cannot complete block designs or copy a complex figure. Such inabilities may be due to apraxia or planning deficits or to problems with spatial relationships. Similarly, it is not always clear whether a memory-impaired patient's deficit is primarily one of impaired attention, poor consolidation or retrieval difficulties.

8.1 TREATMENT MODELS IN REHABILITATION

A theoretical model can be regarded as a representation which may help to explain and increase our understanding of related phenomena. Models vary in complexity and detail, ranging from highly complex computer-based structures, programmed to enable prediction of, say, the weather or the economic situation, to simple analogies which assist in the explanation of relatively complex situations. Thus, for example, in the latter case, Baddeley (1984) uses the analogy of cataloguing in a library to help explain how information is stored in the memory.

In rehabilitation, models are useful for facilitating thinking about treatment, explaining treatment to therapists and relatives, and enabling us to conceptualize outcomes. Gross and Schutz (1986) offer the following five models to assist examination and explanation of treatment within neuropsychology:

1. the environmental control model
2. the stimulus-reponse (S-R) conditioning model
3. the skill training model
4. the strategy substitution model
5. the cognitive cycle model

They claim that these models are hierarchical so that patients who cannot learn are treated with environmental control techniques; patients who can learn but cannot generalize need S–R conditioning; patients who can learn and generalize but cannot self-monitor should be given skill training; those who can self-monitor will benefit from strategy substitution; and those who can manage all of the above and are able to set their own goals will be best suited for treatment that is incorporated within the cognitive cycle model.

Although such a hierarchical model has a neatness about it, a rigid adherence to its parameters could lead to some spurious conclusions. It is highly unlikely, for example, that absolute agreement would be found between therapists who were asked to make decisions about whether a particular patient could learn or generalize. These models imply that an inability to learn can be recognized with relative ease, yet we know that even comatose head-injured patients are capable of some degree of learning (Boyle and Green, 1983). Furthermore, it is possible to teach generalization in some instances (Zarkowska, 1987). Despite these, and possibly other reservations, it can be argued that Gross and Schutz's models are useful in encouraging therapists to think about ways of tackling problems arising from severe head injury.

Powell (1981) outlines six paradigms or models of treatment:

1. The non-intervention strategy (letting nature take its course);
2. The prosthetic paradigm whereby patients are helped to make the most effective use of prostheses;
3. Practice or stimulation, which is probably the most widely used treatment technique, although there is little evidence to support the notion that, on its own, it is effective for many of the problems following severe head injury (Miller, 1984);

4. The maximizing paradigm in which therapists tend to maximize the extent, speed and level of learning by such procedures as positive reinforcement and feedback;
5. Brain function therapy, or directed stimulation which aims to focus or direct tasks at certain regions of the brain to increase its activity or re-establish functions in new areas;
6. Medical, biochemical and surgical treatments which, although beyond the brief of this chapter, can sometimes be combined with other therapeutic treatments (Durand, 1982, for example).

With the exception of medical, biochemical and surgical models, the others described by Gross and Schutz (1986) and Powell (1981) can be classified as belonging to one or other of the disciplines of neuro-psychology, cognitive and behavioural psychology. These disciplines can be drawn upon to inform much of what goes on in rehabilitation, and this is particularly so in the case of treatment for cognitive impair-ment. For example, the principles and techniques of neuro-psychological assessment enable us to diagnose the presence or absence of such cognitive deficits as unilateral visual neglect or prosopagnosia. Localization models help us to understand certain aspects of the organization of the brain so that in cases of focal lesions it might be possible to achieve goals by using the abilities of its non-damaged areas. For example, people who have verbal memory deficits following left hemisphere damage can be taught or encouraged to remember by turning verbal tasks into visual ones, thus encouraging remembering by using the intact right hemisphere. This is likely to be difficult for the traumatically brain-injured, however, where widespread, diffuse damage is the norm.

The study of specific diagnostic groups such as post-encephalitic patients, or those who have undergone hemispherectomy operations may help us plan treatment and predict outcome to a limited extent although, once again, as far as people with head injury are concerned there is a particular lack of homogeneity. Nevertheless, it is likely that recovery continues for much longer than is the case with other diagnostic groups.

Probably the biggest potential contribution of neuropsychology lies in the identification of underlying concepts of the nature of brain damage and how this might reflect on the response to rehabilitation or the selection of appropriate treatment strategies. For example, if it could be demonstrated that repair of tissue damage was possible by specific stimulation procedures during a critical period then we could engineer the introduction of rehabilitation to maximize this repair. At present, however, it is probably fair to say that although neuropsychology is helpful in identifying and specifying deficits, it has not yet had a major influence on the treatment of those deficits.

Aspects of cognitive psychology have informed our diagnosis and conceptualization of disorders such as dyslexia and amnesia. The dual-route model of reading (Coltheart, 1985), for example, has not only proved useful in distinguishing between surface and phonological dyslexia but has also been offered as an explanation for the success of certain reading remediation programmes. Wilson (1987) describes two head-injured people who became almost totally alexic following their accidents. Both were taught to read again although, following treatment, they showed characteristics of surface dyslexia where the most striking feature was a difficulty in reading irregular words. Thus it appeared that one of the dual routes (the phonological route) was accessible, or could be redeveloped, although the other (the lexical or whole-word route) was not.

Models of human memory and theoretical interpretations of the human amnesic syndrome have also been provided by cognitive psychologists. Both these areas have contributed to the diagnosis and understanding of memory deficits. Distinctions made by cognitive psychologists between semantic, episodic and procedural memory have influenced the way we conceptualize disorders. Explanations of encoding, storage and retrieval deficits have influenced assessment techniques (Wilson, 1987, for a further discussion).

In terms of treatment, however, cognitive psychology, like neuropsychology, has not featured strongly in rehabilitation. There are some exceptions – particularly in the field of memory therapy where techniques based upon models of visual imagery have been adopted in memory therapy programmes (for example, Crovitz et al., 1979; Glasgow et al., 1977; Jones, 1974; Wilson and Moffat, 1984a; b). The method of expanding rehearsal or distributed practice, described by Landauer and Bjork (1978), has also been applied in rehabilitation when one piece of information is presented to a patient who is then tested immediately, tested again after a short delay, again after a slightly longer delay and so forth.

One of the phenomena which interested cognitive psychologists working in the field of amnesia was that people with the amnesic syndrome could learn certain tasks or skills relatively well. These included motor skills as demonstrated by a pursuit-rotor task (Brooks and Baddeley, 1976), jigsaw assembly tasks (Brooks and Baddeley, 1976), eyelid conditioning (Weiskrantz and Warrington, 1979), perceptual learning (Williams, 1953; Warrington and Weiskrantz, 1968), certain paired-associates (Warrington and Weiskrantz, 1982), and a rule for solving a complex puzzle (Cohen and Corkin, 1981). The learning of these tasks is usually described as procedural learning. Baddeley (1982) suggests that the feature shared by all these tasks is that subjects have to show learning by actually demonstrating the task; it is not necessary for them to be aware of having encountered the material previously.

At first sight it looks as if procedural learning could play a significant part in memory rehabilitation but in fact its role so far has been slight. This is likely to be due to the fact that therapists have not capitalized on this intact area of ability found in many of their amnesic patients. Schacter and Glisky (1986) went some way towards this in an attempt to teach computer skills to memory-impaired people. They noted that some amnesics possess intact skill learning abilities and that these same people benefit from direct priming.

Priming occurs when a single exposure to an item such as a word facilitates performance on a test that does not require conscious recollection. An example of this would be the presentation of a word, say, 'chemical', and a later presentation of a fragment of the word, such as 'ch'. The subject is asked to complete the word with the first word that comes to mind. Priming is said to have occurred if the subject responds with the word provided initially. (Baddeley, 1982, includes this task under the heading of procedural learning.) Schacter and Glisky (1986) then proceeded to teach their amnesic subjects a series of computer programming tasks. They taught them using a method they named 'the method of vanishing cues' whereby the cue to complete each stage of the task is gradually reduced or faded out one letter at a time. Subjects were more successful learning the tasks this way than in a repetitive drill procedure.

However, quite apart from the fact that the 'method of vanishing cues' is very similar to several procedures from behavioural psychology (shaping, chaining, prompting and fading) which have been in existence for a number of years, it is not clear that procedural learning or priming was the explanation for success. The characteristic feature of procedural learning is that amnesic patients succeed although they are unaware of having been previously presented with the material. Schacter and Glisky's subjects took many trials to learn the tasks even with the 'method of vanishing cues'. This is unlike the preserved learning skills described in amnesic patients. On the other hand, when the tasks were learned the subjects were unable to describe *what* they had learned or *how* they had learned despite being able to demonstrate learning on the computer itself. In this sense the learning could be described as procedural learning.

Apart from memory rehabilitation there has been little in the way of treatment models from cognitive psychology and this has been due to the absence of a good cognitive model of learning. The situation could change with the implementation of parallel distributed processing models referred to earlier. Increasing links between cognitive psychology, behavioural psychology, animal studies, neurophysiology and neuropsychology may have important implications in the future for general principles of rehabilitation. Currently, however, cognitive psychology offers models for analysis rather than models for rehabilitation.

The major contribution from behavioural psychology has been the provision of treatment techniques. Behaviour therapy and behaviour modification have generated a technology of learning based on careful observation and concerned with the gradual increment of appropriate behaviours or the decrement of inappropriate behaviours. This technology lends itself well to rehabilitation. Inherent in the behavioural approach is a commitment to the measurement of treatment effectiveness. The combination of measurement and treatment has produced powerful techniques such as single case experimental designs which are able to evaluate the effectiveness of rehabilitation. They are able to tease out whether improvement has been due to natural recovery or to intervention and therapeutic strategies (Gianutsos and Gianutsos, 1987, for a review of single case designs in rehabilitation).

At a pragmatic level it is likely that behavioural psychology has contributed most to the remediation of cognitive deficits, but the theory underlying the behavioural approach is not impressive. Nevertheless, at a technological level, much has been gained by the application of basic methods to contexts where immediate feedback occurs.

Behavioural psychologists, when faced with a choice between strict adherence to theory such as that laid down by Skinner or Wolpe, and reshaping behavioural models in order to solve problems, have opted pragmatically for the latter. This has resulted in a technology which has replaced fanatical acceptance of a theory. It can be argued that in behavioural psychology the technology has outstripped theory. In the short term this looks as though it has been advantageous because of its practical strengths: things get done and changes occur. However, a technology which moves too far away from its theoretical principles and models is in danger of becoming sterile.

8.2 THE SINFONIA HEMISPHERICA MODEL

If it is true that the discipline which has brought most progress in cognitive rehabilitation is also the one that, in its application to rehabilitation, has strayed furthest from its principles, theoretical frameworks or models, then an impasse is likely to occur, if indeed it has not occurred already. Is there a solution to this dilemma? It would seem that a possible way forward is to think in terms of an overriding 'grand' model for cognitive rehabilitation which combines all three disciplines of neuropsychology, cognitive psychology and behavioural psychology. The model can be refined by thinking of it as one which offers a behavioural technology that is informed by cognitive psychology in order to investigate neuropsychological and neurophysiological issues.

In order to illustrate and perhaps clarify some of the points this model raises we shall refer to an analogy developed by Buffery and Burton (1982). From their analogy it is possible to derive at least four models of cognitive rehabilitation, and from our examination of these we can ask how far each of them fits into our 'grand' model.

Buffery and Burton compared the brain to a symphony orchestra ('Sinfonia Hemispherica'), and brain damage to the situation which might arise should several violinists from the orchestra develop food poisoning and die a few hours before a concert. In this situation the following factors will affect the overall performance of the orchestra:

1. The *size* of the lesion – the more violinists who have died the worse will be the performance;
2. The *position* of the lesion – some violinists, such as the leader, are more important than others;
3. *Shock* – although the remaining members of the orchestra are not ill themselves, initially they will be affected by the sudden demise of their colleagues.

Buffery and Burton suggest several ways the orchestra might cope with its predicament. First, the orchestra could recruit new members to replace those who have died. Second, the orchestra could change its repertoire so that missing members are not required to perform. Third, the leader of the orchestra could ask some other members to learn the violin. These members would not be starting from scratch because they would be able to read music and follow the conductor. However, the subsequent decrease in the number of other instruments would lead to an overall decline in the orchestra's performance. Fourth, the leader could ask other instrumentalists to play the violin parts on their instruments. The resulting sound would not be perfect but would probably be reasonably acceptable. (In all of these alter- natives we are assuming a sympathetic audience who will make allowances for the orchestra's predicament.) How might these alternatives work out in terms of performance, practice and effect? Let us consider them in further detail within a context of cognitive rehabilitation.

Recruiting new or replacement members

Substituting brain for orchestra, this would be equivalent to restoring or repairing damaged tissue. Finger and Stein (1982) describe several ways this might be achieved, including regeneration, diaschisis and plasticity. The last-named involves anatomical reorganization so consideration of this will be postponed until discussion of the third option. Regeneration in the central nervous system (CNS) may occur in a very limited way, an example being the sprouting of axons, but from a functional, behavioural and clinically relevant viewpoint there is no evidence that regeneration within the CNS is a viable outcome of treatment. Diaschisis is a term coined by Von Monakow (1914: translated by Pribam, 1969). It assumes that following damage to the brain, neural shock can occur elsewhere in the brain. Miller (1984) states that:

> the parts of the brain susceptible to this shock effect can be adjacent to the site of the primary insult or in quite distant parts that are linked in some way to the area of primary disturbance. (p. 58)

This concept is similar but not identical to Luria's (1963) theory of inhibition. The major difference is that diaschisis is presumed to travel along specific pathways while inhibition is more diffuse, and affects the brain as a whole. These are the concepts Buffery and Burton (1982) had in mind when they stated that the surviving members of the orchestra would be affected by shock at the death of their violinist colleagues.

Miller (1984) reviews the evidence in favour of diaschisis and finds it unconvincing. Luria's notion of inhibition, however, has led to the development of treatment strategies. His hypothesis was that following brain lesions, primary damage occurred as a result of the death of neurons and secondary damage occurred due to the inhibition of intact neurons. Furthermore, Luria believed that it was possible to de-inhibit these neurons by combining drug treatment with careful training procedures. Drugs would modify poor synaptic transmission and careful training could allow the patient to use residual abilities which could then be substituted for the original, habitual way of performing.

Luria's careful training procedures are very similar to shaping procedures from behaviour therapy. Luria et al. (1969), for example, describes Perelman's work with post-concussional deaf patients. These patients were asked to read sentences which were, at the same time, read aloud by a therapist. Gradually the sentences were written less and less clearly with the pronunciation, on the other hand, remaining perfectly clear. Those patients who possessed inhibited hearing were gradually guided by the sound of the sentence, even when the written version became illegible. What we do not know from Luria's work, however, is how far the patients would have improved without their special training. It is possible that attempts to restore lost functioning can be achieved (or hastened) through deinhibition provided that deficits are the result of secondary rather than primary brain damage. Thus, such approaches would fall into what Miller (1984) describes as artifact theories as explanations of recovery, that is, recovery follows temporary or largely temporary disturbances.

The manner in which such disturbances are resolved, however, is usually far from clear in cognitive rehabilitation programmes which appear to be based on this approach. Apart from the kind of techniques described by Luria et al. (1969), most programmes give the impression that restoration of function is expected to occur through the practice or stimulation of impaired cognitive skills. These are among the most widely used techniques in cognitive rehabilitation, and most computer training programmes are based on these principles. Patients are given practice in programmes aimed at training attention or perception, or re-training memory. Tasks are usually graded from easy to more complex and there is little doubt that most people improve their performance on the tasks themselves. However, there is little evidence that these approaches actually lead to improved performance in attention, perception or memory in other activities connected with daily living (Schacter and Glisky, 1986).

The same criticism can be made of these techniques when they are employed in non-computer-based treatment programmes. Miller (1984) suggests that although most speech therapy programmes attempt to stimulate language, there is insufficient evidence to support the idea that such stimulation is better than spontaneous recovery. Schacter and Glisky (1986), discussing memory therapy programmes state that: '. . . there is no evidence that they [repetitive exercises] can produce a general improvement of mnemonic function in amnesic patients' (p. 260).

Harris and Sunderland (1981) conducted a survey of the management of memory disorders in rehabilitation units in Britain. They found that games and exercises were the most widely used treatment techniques yet no evidence could be obtained to suggest that such pursuits led to improvements in memory functioning. When studies are reported claiming success for approaches involving exercise, stimulation or practice it is usually difficult to separate treatment effectiveness from spontaneous recovery (Miller, 1984, for further discussion).

Obviously, some practice is required in all cognitive programmes but we are still waiting for evidence to support the hypothesis that practice alone will lead to real improvement. On the other hand, we do have evidence that practice alone does *not* produce improvement. For example, Wilson (1982) gave 6 weeks of intensive memory training, exercises and stimulation to a patient with amnesia who, at the end of the programme, showed no improvement at all in general memory functioning. Schacter and Glisky (1986) gave a 2-hour memory stimulation session for several months to patients who also showed no improvement in their general level of memory functioning at the end of the course.

Another question concerning the exercise/stimulation model involves generalization. It has been noted frequently that brain-injured people have great difficulty in transferring a solution that works in one situation or for one particular problem, to another situation or problem. It is sometimes argued that computers are useful in rehabilitation because they do not suffer from short-term fatigue, they are reliable, and patients enjoy working on the programmes. If this is the case then therapists need to devise ways to ensure that any improvement on a computer task generalizes to other situations and other behaviours. To return to Buffery and Burton's analogy for a moment, it would be no use if the orchestra leader employed new violinists who could play well in private but could not perform in front of an audience.

Given the major learning and generalization difficulties experienced by our patients, perhaps we should avoid creating a stage which requires transferring skills in a limited clinical context to situations that occur in the 'real world'. Would it not be better to start on the real life skills themselves? This is not to say that computers should be abandoned for assessment and research purposes, nor is it the case that training programmes cannot be devised which avoid the difficulties described above. It is nevertheless difficult to find evidence supporting the efficacy of exercise, practice or stimulation, when these are the only strategies involved in a rehabilitation programme. This holds true for computer training packages as well as for cognitive rehabilitation programmes in general.

To what extent does this model combine elements of the three disciplines we mentioned earlier? Essentially, it is a neuropsychological model concerned with neural regeneration. It asks questions about the nature of brain damage and the replacement of damaged tissues. From references to the work of Luria and his colleagues we find some overlapping dependence upon behavioural techniques (although they are not described as such). However, the predominant treatment procedures are not behavioural, there is little in the way of task analysis, specification of goals, functional analysis, reinforcement, shaping, chaining or modelling. It is obvious, too, that this model owes little to cognitive psychology.

Changing the repertoire so that missing members are not required

In terms of cognitive rehabilitation, this is equivalent to brain-injured people changing their lifestyles in order to avoid problem areas. The model is indistinguishable from the environmental control model disseminated by Gross and Schutz (1986), and referred to above. The origin of the model is to be found within the discipline of behaviour modification. Murphy (1987) states that restructuring the environment is a useful procedure for decreasing undesirable behaviour. She explains that the operant view of behaviour is that it is determined both by consequences and by antecedents. Thus, if it becomes clear that undesirable behaviour occurs only in one situation, it may be possible to modify the situation to prevent the behaviour occurring. This can be an extremely effective and rapid way of eradicating or reducing such behaviours but it is not always possible to do this. Furthermore, it could also be the case that the new, modified environment is, in itself, undesirable. For example, we could keep a patient in hospital where his/her day is structured and no demands are made on memory. This would avoid many of the problems resulting from memory impairment such as getting lost in the neighbourhood, forgetting to pass on messages, and failing to remember an appointment. On the other hand, it might be better to accept these failures than to limit the patient to the expensive, understimulating environment of the hospital ward.

Gross and Schutz (1986) say of the environmental control model that it may 1. serve to prompt adaptive behaviours, 2. make incomplete responses more adequate, and 3. suppress problematic behaviours.

Environmental control is a sensible strategy to use with patients who have severe general intellectual deterioration or several cognitive problems such as difficulty in attending, perceiving and remembering. Probably the best known approach incorporating environmental changes is **reality orientation** with its use of labels, signposts and noticeboards. In this approach the environment is structured so that cognitive demands are reduced for cognitively impaired clients. Colour-coding is another way of achieving this end, and so, too, is the positioning of material or information so that it cannot be missed, ignored or forgotten. This approach can provide instantaneous success. For the patient who cannot remember where the lavatory is, or who keeps getting into the wrong bed, labels and signposts can solve the problem immediately. The patient who neglects one half of space and fails to see the tablets placed on one side of the plate, or indeed ignores the food on that half of the plate, can be helped by having the tablets placed on the opposite side, and all the food pushed to the observable side of the plate. This approach is not always recommended for patients with unilateral neglect and, indeed, it is contrary to current rehabilitation practice (Weinberg et al., 1979; Diller, 1980, for example). Many patients with neglect are not in rehabilitation programmes, however, and sometimes they receive almost no stimulation at all, either through their good or neglected side; and for these patients, particularly when we want to maximize the quality of response (such as taking a personal history or when there has been a poor response to rehabilitation) then re-positioning of material should be considered.

Environmental changes do not, of course, always work. The patient with severe bilateral frontal lobe damage described by Baddeley and Wilson (1988) is a case in point. There were signs and notices all over the rehabilitation centre aimed at reducing the cognitive load on this man. For example, there was a large notice on the way out of the canteen saying, 'Roger, you are in Room 3 after tea', and another sign on the door leading out of the building where Roger's therapy took place, saying, 'Roger, you have gone too far.' But Roger ignored all the signs. He frequently saw and read them but could not alter his response accordingly.

Environmental modifications reduce the cognitive load on brain-injured patients. This can, of course, be achieved in other ways. Thus, instead of asking a patient to remember two or three exercises in physiotherapy, we can ask that patient to remember *one* of those exercises. Instead of asking the patient to read through Chapter One of a computer manual we can ask that patient to read the first page, or even the first paragraph. Sometimes rewording questions can avoid problems. In occupational therapy, for example, instead of saying, 'What exercises would you like to work on today?' to a patient with problems making decisions, we can say, 'Would you prefer to do typing or printing this morning?'

Many cognitive problems are made worse by anxiety, fatigue and stress, or by distractions from the environment. Thus, a patient who has difficulty in concentrating may perform much better alone in a room than with a number of people present. Obviously, it is not always practical or desirable to work in a one-to-one situation, but it might be better to begin in this way, perhaps by putting a screen around the patient and the immediate work area, then gradually exposing more distracting stimuli. Gross and Schutz (1986) give the example of a head-injured client who was having difficulties in settling back into her work because she was easily distracted. The employer was instructed to minimize distracting stimuli in the client's vicinity by moving the workbench to a relatively secluded part of the workshop and by instructing her colleagues not to engage in conversation with her during work hours.

Changing the repertoire or bypassing and thus avoiding problem areas through environmental restructuring is a fruitful treatment strategy, particularly with the severely intellectually impaired. There is evidence for its effectiveness. Two studies with the confused elderly, for example, showed that patients were able to learn to find their way around the hospital ward when clear signposting was used (Hanley, 1981; Gilleard et al., 1981). Such an approach is primarily behavioural, using the technique of environmental restructuring, a well established procedure in behaviour modification. It is also analagous to Powell's maximizing paradigm in which a person's best responses are maximized through a therapist's response.

There is some indirect influence from cognitive psychology in this treatment in so far as it is concerned with reducing the cognitive demands made on the individual and thus it could be classified as an information processing model. It should be possible, however, to expand the influences of both cognitive and neuropsychology to tailor this approach to those cognitive capacities that are absent and those that remain.

Ask other members of the orchestra to learn the violin

In cognitive rehabilitation this is equivalent to anatomical reorganization which is based on the idea that undamaged areas of the brain can take on the skills or functions subserved by a damaged area. It differs from the regrowth in the CNS model described above in that anatomical reorganization implies that a *different* part of the brain is encouraged to take over from the part originally used for a particular skill or function. The regrowth or regeneration model seeks to restore the original, damaged area.

Anatomical reorganization is a controversial approach to rehabilitation although belief in its efficacy appears to be widely accepted by relatives and the general public. We have frequently heard the view from families of brain-injured people that humans only use a small percentage of their brain and that large areas are unused or untapped. Unfortunately, myths are sometimes made to look like facts when spurious data is attached to them by people in the media (for example, MccGwuire (1986): 'We make use of only 10 per cent of our brains . . .' (p. 85).

Miller (1984) discussed the idea of anatomical reorganization in some detail. He comes to the conclusion that:

> anatomical reorganization in some form can and does occur in the very young. The status of this principle as an explanation of recovery in mature subjects is much more open to question. (p. 67)

Cases where anatomical reorganization is a convincing explanation for recovery of function are due to the potential for cerebral plasticity in immature organisms. We mentioned earlier that Finger and Stein (1982) put plasticity forward as one model of recovery.

The most convincing evidence for plasticity comes from studies of infants who have had their left cerebral hemisphere removed in early life and who have then gone on to develop language in the right hemisphere (Kohn and Dennis, 1978, for example). In such cases this language development could mean 1. that one structure (that is, the right hemisphere) has taken over the functions of another (the left hemisphere), or 2. that the right hemisphere has strengthened previously weak and ineffective connections/pathways/abilities. Finger and Stein call this latter procedure 'supersensitivity'. We know from the work of researchers such as Searleman (1977) and Zaidel (1977) that the right hemisphere in adults has some language ability. Witelson (1977) believes that the right hemisphere has a greater role in speech and language functions in children than it does in adults, so it could well be that the supersensitivity principle is operating – at least in cases of language reorganization. However, even though anatomical reorganization indubitably takes place in the very young, it may be at the expense of other abilities (Dennis and Kohn, 1975), or be incomplete. In the words of Byrne and Gates (1987):

> despite substantial development of ability systems normally subserved by the removed hemisphere, very subtle limitations of ability development were evident, suggesting in fact a degree of hemispheric functional specificity. (p. 424)

In the case of the adult brain-injured population few treatments are implemented with the specific aim of encouraging anatomical reorganization. An exception is a method known as brain function therapy. Buffery (1976) was probably the first to use this term. He describes a patient with aphasia following a left hemisphere stroke. Buffery attempted to stimulate the right cerebral hemisphere through tachistoscopic presentation and through auditory and tactile stimuli. He wanted to encourage language to develop in the right hemisphere. The patient showed some improvement and Buffery claimed this was evidence that the right hemisphere became better at handling verbal material. However, other explanations are possible. An equally valid explanation is that the information going into the right hemisphere was passed across the corpus collosum into the left hemisphere and that the improvement in language functioning was due to improvement in the functioning of the left hemisphere.

We should conclude, at this stage in the search for evidence, that the case remains unproven. It is certain that there are no studies available to us that demonstrate that undamaged parts of the brain can take over the functions of the damaged parts in adults surviving severe head injury. As far as Buffery's analogy is concerned, the oboe and trumpet players will not be able to switch to playing the violin. Again, the model we have discussed in this section is predominantly neuropsychological. Given the unlikelihood of this model being viable in cognitive rehabilitation, we do not need to reflect upon possible influences from the fields of cognitive and behavioural psychology.

Ask other instrumentalists to learn the violin parts

In cognitive rehabilitation terms, this possibility is equivalent to functional adaptation (finding the next best solution). This approach appears to be one of the most successful in rehabilitation, with its underlying principle of urging therapists to look for alternative solutions that will enable the patient to achieve success at a task that cannot now be solved in the usual manner. Functional adaptation has been shown to occur in animals. Finger and Stein (1982) describe how rats with locomotor problems following medial parietal lesions can be taught to run at the same speed as they achieved prior to the operation. The pattern of movements used to achieve this, however, was different. Luria et al. (1969) discuss functional adaptations along with other ideas about restoration of function. They believe that these functional adaptations are much more important from the clinical point of view than either anatomical reorganization or deinhibition. (The reader is referred to the 1969 paper for expansion of Luria's ideas on functional adaptation.)

A host of aids for activities of daily living can be described as functional adaptations: for example, velcro fastenings for people who cannot manage zips or buttons, and long handled picking-up sticks for those who cannot bend down. In cognitive rehabilitation, too, there are a number of alternative solutions we can employ. External memory aids such as tape recorders, computers, notebooks and databank wristwatches are examples of the use of prosthetic memory amongst those whose natural powers of remembering no longer match the demands made upon them. Miller (1984), for example, describes a clerk who was unable to remember what information to request from customers. The clerk was helped by providing him with a specially designed notepad. Each sheet of the notepad contained a duplicated outline of the information to be extracted from each customer.

Examples of other alternative solutions are:

1. Canon communicators (calculator-sized machines on which messages can be typed and printed out on ticker tape) that can be employed by those who have severe speech difficulties in the presence of intact language skills;
2. Reading through tactile impressions (tracing letters with a finger) when reading by vision is impossible (Landis et al. (1982) and Wilson (1986), for examples);
3. Using symbolic language systems such as Amerind (Skelly, 1979) or Visual Communication in Aphasia (VIC – Gardner et al., 1976) for the severely language impaired. Wilson (1986) gives an example of such a system with a globally aphasic stroke patient. The subject was unable to utter even one word and his comprehension was at a 2-year-old level. Nevertheless, a simple, alternative communication system was established through the use of visual symbols.

Functional adaptation is similar to a behavioural approach to treatment. Both are more concerned with achieving goals than with the mechanisms by which these goals are reached. Miller (1984) states that:

> of the processes that might be invoked to explain longer-term recovery in mature subjects functional adaptation or compensation is the only one that can be regarded as having definitely been shown to occur under at least some circumstances. (pp. 76-77).

The question as to whether such compensation occurs spontaneously or only after special training remains unanswered.

This model comes closest to combining influences, in the form of theoretical background and methodologies, from all three disciplines of neuropsychology, cognitive psychology and behavioural psychology. Precise identification of neuropsychological strengths and weaknesses are required in order to ascertain why a patient has a memory deficit or reading difficulty or language problem. Reference to neuropsychology is required in order to bypass weaknesses caused by brain injury and select possible alternative areas of the brain that are undamaged. Cognitive psychology can provide us with certain techniques for achieving goals in different ways. Thus, for example, visual imagery can be used to enable people to remember verbal material. From a more theoretical level we can sometimes take models of cognitive functioning to help us design alternative ways of reaching goals. The dual route model of reading, for example, (Coltheart, 1985) proposes that we can read by using a whole-word lexical route or by using a phonological rule based route. When people become dyslexic following brain damage it is sometimes possible to teach them to read again through the use of the unimpaired or less damaged route. Behavioural psychology provides us with the means to identify the everyday implications or manifestations of cognitive deficits as well as the means to teach people how to achieve goals in alternative ways.

8.3 LIMITATIONS OF THE SINFONIA HEMISPHERICA MODEL

Buffery and Burton's (1982) model does not take into account the situation which usually occurs in head injury, namely that isolated focal lesions rarely occur. Widespread, diffuse damage is much more likely so the orchestra would not lose *all* the violinists, nor would it lose *only* violinists. Thus, as far as cognitive rehabilitation for the traumatically brain-injured is concerned, models which assume all-or-none damage are limited as most patients will sustain multiple, partial lesions.

It is possible that the recent parallel distributed processing models (Hinton and Anderson, 1981; Rumelhart and McClelland, 1986) will be more appropriate for the head-injured population. One of the characteristics of these models is to explain deficits following structural damage as 'graceful degradation'. Current explanations of cognitive deficits are beginning to be influenced by these models (see Patterson, Seidenburg and McClelland, in press).

To return to the Sinfonia Hemispherica analogy, if the violinists are reduced in number and the surviving members are functioning poorly, then it might be possible to enable the remaining players to make more efficient use of their surviving skills. It is likely that in at least some instances of cognitive rehabilitation with the head-injured, success has been achieved because the rehabilitation procedures employed by therapists have enabled the brain-injured to use their residual skills more effectively.

Sometimes this can be done by making sure people allow themselves extra time to learn new information. They can be taught to organize information or make associations between that which they already know and that which they are trying to learn. Mnemonics, for example, probably work because they allow previously isolated items to become integrated with one another (Bower, 1972). It is possible to teach some memory-impaired people to use a mnemonic system to help them learn better. One young man, for example, was taught the face-name association procedure (McCarty, 1980) to enable him to learn people's names. He worked part-time in his father's jeweller's shop and adapted the face-name method not to remember names but to remember which person he had been serving when he went to get something out of the window display. He would, for instance, say under his breath, 'Mr Puffy Face' or 'Mrs Red Eyes'.

Another method which appears to work because it enables head-injured people to use impoverished memory skills more efficiently is the PQRST method. This is an acronym for Preview, Question, Read, State and Test, first reported by Robinson (1970). Wilson (1987) compared PQRST with rote rehearsal for recall of verbal material. Eight head-injured patients took part and each was seen individually on six occasions. On these occasions two stories were presented, one of which required subjects to use rote rehearsal and one required them to use the PQRST. The order of presentation was balanced across subjects and presentations. An equal amount of time was spent on each story. Subjects were tested for immediate and delayed recall and for the percentage of information retained after a delay. In the delayed recall condition and in the percentage of information retained the PQRST method was significantly superior to rote recall.

Another variation on this theme is to teach people to compensate for certain cognitive impairments by capitalizing on their cognitive strengths. Examples of this can be seen fairly often in right hemisphere stroke patients who have difficulty in topographical orientation. They know that they have difficulty finding their way around *spatially*, but they are as good as ever *verbally*. One way forward for such people is to make efforts to turn spatial tasks into verbal ones. One man, for example, reported that he could never find his way to the ward until he told himself to look for the door near the 'no-entry' road sign. Once he had verbalized this spatial task he was always able to find the ward.

Methods for teaching the cognitively impaired to use their existing skills more efficiently can be found in both cognitive and behavioural psychology techniques. Chunking, organization and rehearsal techniques such as Landauer and Bjork's method of expanding rehearsal (1978) are all potentially useful. PQRST was one of the procedures described in *Effective Study* by Robinson (1970). It is possible that

PQRST is superior to rote rehearsal because it involves deeper levels of processing. The levels of processing model (Craik and Lockhart, 1972) states that the deeper material is processed the better it is remembered. In the PQRST method subjects have to think about the material they are reading or listening to in order to complete each of the stages whereas in rote rehearsal they simply need to listen and repeat back.

Mnemonics, also from the field of cognitive psychology, probably enable people to make better use of existing skills. Bower (1972) suggests that mnemonics allow previously isolated items to become integrated with one another. If we can help head-injured people to do this and thus enable them to learn information more effectively, then we are helping them to make more efficient use of existing skills.

From behaviour therapy and behaviour modification have come other techniques to aid in this approach. Goodkin (1966), for example, used operant conditioning to improve handwriting in a patient with Parkinson's disease; Wilson (1981) described how modelling was employed to improve communication in a globally aphasic stroke patient. Behaviour modification programmes, used traditionally to decrease undesirable behaviours, have provided a valuable structure for the design of cognitive rehabilitation programmes, including those which enable head-injured people to use existing skills more efficiently. (See Wilson, in press, for an example of this method with an apraxic man who had difficulty writing letters of the alphabet.)

This approach is another which combines theoretical background and methodological approaches from all three disciplines of neuro-psychology, cognitive psychology and behavioural psychology. The specification of neuropsychological strengths and weaknesses is essential if we are to know *what* can and cannot be achieved and *why*. Cognitive psychology not only provides some strategies but should also enable us to understand and explain why somebody cannot read, write, interpret visual material or whatever. Once again, behavioural assessment and treatment techniques provide a structure and a means for monitoring and evaluating the effectiveness of intervention.

In summarizing this section it would be true to say that, given our present stage of development in the field of cognitive rehabilitation, the most fruitful approaches are those which attempt to 1. find alternative solutions, or 2. bypass the problem areas, or 3. find ways to use existing skills more efficiently.

8.4 CONCLUDING REMARKS

The approaches to cognitive rehabilitation described above should not be regarded as mutually exclusive. In fact, several, if not all, of them may be useful in a treatment programme, either at different stages of recovery or for different cognitive problems experienced by a particular patient. Indeed, some may be used simultaneously for treatment of a single problem. Using more than one approach makes sense because we cannot afford to reject ideas which might help some of our patients, and we know that using dual coding or two routes to tackle the same problem can be more efficient than relying on one. This is consistent with Paivio's (1971) dual route theory, and is discussed in Wilson (1987).

In conclusion, I would like to refer to the treatment of a young woman who sustained a very severe head injury in a horse riding accident. I have selected out this example because it serves the purpose of focusing most of the points I have been making in this chapter, and because it illustrates that progress in cognitive rehabilitation can be made based on treatment that is organized, monitored and evaluated. Among other cognitive problems, this young woman lost completely the ability to read. A programme was designed, and has been described by Wilson and Baddeley (1986) and Wilson (1987). Initially, we retaught her the letters of the alphabet, one at a time. Learning was very slow: for example, she took 6 weeks to learn the letter 'y'. After 9 months she had relearned all 26 letters and was then taught several more complex rules, such as how to pronounce 'igh' and 'wr'. Eventually, she was reading at the level of an 11-year-old. During treatment, most of the cognitive rehabilitation approaches described above were introduced, as can be seen in Table 8.2.

It should be stressed that cognitive rehabilitation is potentially a rewarding field in which to work. Cognitive problems faced by head-injured people are likely to be the most handicapping in the long run, yet there is always something which can be done to help alleviate their everyday problems. It is essential, however, that we ensure that cognitive rehabilitation programmes are properly monitored and evaluated. In this way we can develop and extend this important area, and at the same time avoid shallow answers to important questions. As far as we can tell, there are no quick solutions and 'bandwaggoning' must be resisted. Our attitude towards computer training packages, for instance, should be critically analytical rather than superficially impressionable. As yet, there is no sound evidence that these programmes genuinely help the real-life problems experienced by the cognitively impaired, although there is likely to be an important

Table 8.2 Cognitive rehabilitation approaches for a young woman with severe head injurys following a horse riding accident

Treatment approach	Example
Restoration of function	We wanted to teach the young woman to read again. Exercises and practice played a part in the overall programme.
Environmental changes	Initially, we changed her reading 'environment' by giving her specially prepared material, and by drawing pictures to help her remember.
Brain function therapy	We did not attempt this directly, but anatomical reorganization could have been part of the explanation.
Functional adaptations/ alternative solutions	At the beginning we tried to teach her to become a letter-by-letter reader.
Use of existing skills more efficiently	She knew whether a stimulus was a word or a letter. She was able to use her verbal descriptions of the stimulus: for example, 'An 'O' with a tail is a 'Q'.' Rewards and other strategies from behaviour therapy were incorporated into the treatment programme.

place for them in the future as functional adaptations. The point to stress is that without rigorous recording, monitoring and evaluation, cognitive rehabilitation could become nothing more than a passing fad and go the way of phrenology or sleep-teaching machines. We owe it to the patients to make sure our discipline is properly supported by strong theoretical frameworks, sound research, and detailed scrutiny of practice.

REFERENCES

Baddeley, A.D. (1982) Implications of neuropsychological evidence for theories of normal memory. *Phil. Trans. R. Soc. Lond. B*, **298**, 59-72.

Baddeley, A.D. (1984) Memory theory and memory therapy, in *Clinical Management of Memory Problems* (B. Wilson and N. Moffat, eds), Croom Helm, London; Aspen Publishers, Rockville, MD.

Baddeley, A.D. and Wilson, B.A. (1988) Frontal amnesia and the dysexecutive syndrome. *Brain and Cognition*, **7**, 212-30.

Bower, G.H. (1972) A selective review of organizational factors in memory, in *Organization of Memory* (E. Tulving and W. Donaldson, eds), Academic Press, New York.

Boyle, M.E. and Green, R.D. (1983) Operant procedures and the comatose patient. *J. Appl. Behav. Anal.*, **16**, 3-12.

Brooks, D.N. and Baddeley, A.D. (1976) What can amnesics learn? *Neuropsychologia*, **14**, 111-22.

Buffery, A.W.H. (1976) Clinical neuropsychology: a review and preview, in *Contributions to Medical Psychology* (S. Rachman, ed.), Pergamon Press, Oxford.

Buffery, A.W.H. and Burton, A. (1982) Information processing and redevelopment: towards a science of neuropsychological rehabilitation, in *The Pathology and Psychology of Cognition* (A. Burton, ed), Methuen, London.

Byrne, J.M. and Gates, R.D. (1987) Single-case study of left cerebral hemispherectomy: development in the first five years. *J. Clin. Exper. Neuropsychol.*, **9**, 423-34.

Cohen, N.J. and Corkin, S. (1981) The amnesic patient and retention of a cognitive skill. Paper presented at the *Society for Neuroscience*, Los Angeles, Oct. 1981.

Coltheart, M. (1985) Cognitive neuropsychology and reading, in *Attention and Performance, vol. 11* (M. Posner and O.S.M. Marin, eds), Erlbaum, Hillsdale, NJ.

Craik, F.I.M. and Lockhart, R.S. (1972) Levels of processing: a framework for memory research. *J. Verb. Learn. Verb. Behav.*, **11**, 671-84.

Crovitz, H., Harvey, M. and Horn, R. (1979) Problems in the acquisition of imagery mnemonics: three brain damaged cases. *Cortex*, **15**, 225-34.

Dennis, M. and Kohn, B. (1975) Comprehension of syntax in infantile hemiplegics after cerebral hemidecortication: left hemisphere superiority. *Brain and Language*, **2**, 472-82.

Diller, L. (1980) Development of a perceptual remedial program, in *Behavioural Psychology in Rehabilitation Medicine* (L. Ince, ed.), Williams and Wilkins, Baltimore.

Durand, V.M. (1982) A behavioural/pharmacological intervention for the treatment of severe self-injurious behaviour. *J. Autism Develop. Disord.*, **12**, 243-51.

Finger, S. and Stein, D. (1982) *Brain Damage and Recovery*, Academic Press, New York.

Gardner, H., Zuriff, E.B., Berry, T. and Baker, E. (1976) Visual communication in aphasia. *Neuropsychologia*, **14**, 275-92.

Gianutsos, R. and Gianutsos, J. (1987) Single-case experimental approaches to the assessment of intervention in rehabilitation, in *Rehabilitation Psychology Desk Reference* (B. Caplan, ed) Aspen Publishers, Rockville, MD.

Gilleard, C.J., Mitchell, R.G. and Riordan, J. (1981) Ward orientation training with psychogeriatric patients. *J. Adv. Nurs.*, **6**, 95-98.

Glasgow, R.E., Zeiss, R.A., Barrera, M. and Lewinsohn, P.M. (1977) Case studies on remediating memory deficits in brain damaged individuals. *J. Clin. Psychol.*, **33**, 1049-54.

Goodkin, R. (1966) Case studies in behavioural research in rehabilitation. *Perceptual and Motor Skills*, **23**, 171-82.

Gross, Y. and Schutz, L.E. (1986) Intervention models in neuropsychology, in *Clinical Neuropsychology of Intervention* (B.P. Uzzell and Y. Gross, eds) Martinus Nijhoff, Boston, pp. 179-204.

Hanley, I.G. (1981) The use of signposts and active training to modify ward disorientation in elderly patients. *J. Behav. Ther. Exper. Psychiat.*, **12**, 241-247.

Harris, J.E. and Sunderland, A. (1981) A brief survey of the management of memory disorders in rehabilitation units in Britain. *Int. Rehabil. Med.*, **3**, 206-09.

Hinton, G.E. and Anderson, J.A. (1981) *Parallel Models of Associative Memory*, Erlbaum, Hillsdale, NJ.

Jones, M. (1974) Imagery as a mnemonic aid after left temporal lobectomy: contrast between material specific and generalized memory disorders. *Neuropsychologia*, **12**, 21-30.

Kohn, B. and Dennis, M. (1978) Selective impairments of visuospatial abilities in infantile hemiplegics after right cerebral hemidecortication. *Neuropsychologia*, **12**, 505-12.

Landauer, T.K. and Bjork, R.A. (1978) Optimum rehearsal patterns and name learning, in *Practical Aspects of Memory* (M.M. Gruneberg, P.E. Morris and R.N. Sykes, eds), Academic Press, London.

Landis, T., Graves, R., Benson, D.F. and Hebben, N. (1982) Visual recognition through kinaesthetic mediation. *Psychological Medicine*, **12**, 515-31.

Luria, A.R. (1963) *Recovery of Function After Brain Injury*, Macmillan, New York.

Luria, A.R., Naydin, V.L., Tsvetkova, L.S. and Vinarskaya, E.N. (1969) Restoration of higher cortical function following local brain damage, in *Handbook of Clinical Neurology, vol. 3* (P.J. Vinken and G.W. Bruyn, eds), North Holland, Amsterdam.

McCarty, D. (1980) Investigations of a visual imagery mnemonic device for acquiring face – name associations. *J. Expt. Psychol.*, **6**, 145-55.

MccGwire, S. (1986) *Kim's Story. A Fight for Life*, Harrap, London.

Miller, E. (1984) *Recovery and Management of Neuropsychological Impairments*, John Wiley, Chichester.

Murphy, G. (1987) Decreasing undesirable behaviours, in *Behaviour Modification for People with Mental Handicaps* (W. Yule and J. Carr, eds), Croom Helm, London.

Paivio, A. (1971) *Imagery and Verbal Processes*, Holt, Rinehart and Winston, New York.

Patterson, K., Seidenberg M.S. and McClelland J.L. (in press) Connections and disconnections: acquired dyslexia in a connectionist model of oral reading, in *Parallel Distributed Processing: Implications for Psychology and Neurobiology* (R.G.M. Morris, ed), Oxford University Press.

Powell, G.E. (1981) *Brain Function Therapy*, Gower Press. Aldershot.

Pribham, K.H. (1969) *Brain and Behaviour, 1. Mood States and Mind*, Penguin, Harmondsworth.

Robinson, F.P. (1970) *Effective Study*, Harper & Row, New York.

Rumelhart, D.E. and McClelland, J.L. (1986) *Parallel Distributed Processing: Explorations in the Microstructure of Cognition, Vol. 1*, MIT Press, Cambridge, MA.

Schacter, D.L. and Glisky, E.L. (1986) Memory remediation: restoration, alleviation and the acquisition of domain-specific knowledge, in *Clinical Neuropsychology of Intervention* (B.P. Uzzell and Y. Gross, eds), Martinus Nijhoff, Boston, pp. 257-82.

Searleman, A. (1977) A review of right hemisphere linguistic capabilities. *Psycholog. Bull.*, **84**, 503-28.

Skelly, M. (1979) *Ameri-Ind Gestural Code Based on Universal American Indian Hand Talk*, Elsevier, New York.

Warrington, E.K. and Weiskrantz, L. (1968) New method of testing long-term retention with special reference to amnesic patients. *Nature*, **217**, 972-74.

Warrington, E.K. and Weiskrantz, L. (1982) Amnesia: a disconnection syndrome? *Neuropsychologia*, **20**, 233-248.

Weinberg, J., Diller, L., Gordon, W.A., et al. (1979) Training sensory awareness and spatial organization in people with right brain damage. *Arch. Phys. Med. Rehabil.*, **60**, 491-96.

Weiskrantz, L. and Warrington, E.K. (1979) Conditioning in amnesic patients. *Neuropsychologia*, **17**, 187-94.

Williams, M. (1953) Investigations of amnesic defects by progressive prompting. *J. Neurol., Neurosurg. Psychiat.*, **16**, 14.

Wilson, B.A. (1981) A survey of behavioural treatments carried out at a rehabilitation centre for stroke and head injuries, in *Brain Function Therapy* (G. Powell, ed), Gower Press, Aldershot.

Wilson, B.A. (1982) Success and failure in memory training following a cerebral vascular accident. *Cortex*, **18**, 581-94.

Wilson, B.A. (1986) Cognitive rehabilitation following severe head injury, in *Current Issues in Clinical Psychology* (N. Eisenberg, D. Glasgow, eds).

Wilson, B.A. (1987) *Rehabilitation of Memory*, Guilford Press, New York.

Wilson, B.A. (in press) Cognitive rehabilitation for brain injured adults, in *Traumatic Brain Injury* (B. Deelman, ed.) Swets and Zeitlinger, Lisse, Netherlands.

Wilson, B.A. and Baddeley, A.D. (1986) Single case methodology and the remediation of dyslexia, in *Dyslexia: Neuropsychology and Treatment* (G. Pavlides and D. Fisher, eds), Erlbaum, Hillsdale, NJ.

Wilson, B.A. and Moffat, N. (eds) (1984a) *Clinical Management of Memory Problems*, Croom Helm, London; Aspen Publishers, Rockville, MD.

Wilson, B.A. and Moffat, N. (1984b) Rehabilitation of memory for everyday life, in *Everday Memory: Actions and Absentmindedness* (J. Harris and P. Morris, eds), Academic Press, London.

Witelson, S.F. (1977) Early hemisphere specialisation and interhemispheric plasticity: an empirical and theoretical review, in *Language Development and Neurological Theory* (S.J. Segalowitz and F.A. Gruber, eds) Academic Press, New York, pp. 213-89.

Zaidel, E. (1977) Unilateral auditory language comprehension on the Token Test following commissurotomy and hemispheroctomy. *Neuropsychologia*, **15**, 1-18.

Zarkowska, E. (1987) Discrimination and generalization, in *Behaviour Modification for People with Mental Handicaps*, 2nd edn. (W. Yule and J. Carr, eds) Croom Helm, London.

9   Social rehabilitation: the role of the transitional living centre

Scott Goll and Keith Hawley

Rehabilitation as a service to individuals who have suffered serious head trauma has a relatively short history. Before World War II, most people who sustained severe trauma to the head or spine, if they survived, were sent to acute hospitals and then either to a nursing home or to the family home to be cared for for the rest of their lives. It was not until the end of World War II that the first rehabilitation efforts for the spinal-injured began to take shape. Today there is a developed and rapidly advancing technology in the rehabilitation of individuals with spinal cord injury. Head injury rehabilitation, on the other hand, is just beginning to experience the development of more sophisticated treatment approaches and technologies.

The development of more advanced rehabilitation techniques has its direct roots in the survival rates of people who have sustained a head injury. The current statistics indicate that the survival rate has increased dramatically (National Head Injury Foundation, 1980). In 1966, one out of every two survived a severe trauma to the brain. Today, due to advanced life saving techniques, that number has increased to nine out of ten.

With the increase in the survival of severely head-injured individuals comes the difficult task of rehabilitation. Undoubtedly, medical stability is the essence of early efforts to deal with the effects of trauma to the brain. Early rehabilitation begins as soon as medical stability has been achieved yet acute rehabilitation for the head-injured retains a major medical focus in order to prevent such complications as decubitus ulcers and contractures. Treatment of these problems has been regarded as a prerequisite to achieving and sustaining more substantial goals in the future (Young *et al.*, 1982). As one begins to achieve greater medical stability and make physical progress, the prognosis for the person can look deceptively bright. The injured individual moves into a stage of rehabilitation where cognitive and social issues become more of a focus. These issues will have significant implications for the long-term outcome of the head-injured person.

The purpose of this chapter is to consider a model of rehabilitation which emphasizes the need to help head-injured individuals to adapt successfully to life in the community by using a 'domestic' rather than a 'medical' setting to provide treatment.

During the early years of head injury rehabilitation, a variety of attempts were made to address the long-term social problems of the head-injured. Generally, this meant using an existing system to solve the problem. In most cases, this involved placement in homes for the retarded, community half-way houses for the mentally ill and even psychiatric institutions. Even today, with the increasing awareness of the needs of the head-injured and the extensive development of specialized head injury programmes, inappropriate placement in these types of institution continues to occur.

As professionals and families struggled with the long-term social effects of head injury, it became clearer that the needs of this group were very specialized. By 1970, with a few exceptions, the head-injured and their families were still left to their own resources to pull together some measures of support and intervention to meet the long-term needs. In 1974, Ashby House was established to meet the specific needs of the head-injured. This pioneering effort, located in Toronto, Canada, provided a valuable model for the individuals who would establish programmes in subsequent years. In essence, this **transitional living programme** broke the mould of treatment for the long-term effects of the head-injured.

Interestingly enough, the concept of a transitional living programme did not immediately catch on in the rehabilitation community. Reasons for this included the prevalent requirement to provide 'medically' necessary services in the hospital only, and because of the medically-orientated tradition of rehabilitation, it was not until 1977 that this type of programme began to take hold in the USA. Programmes in the USA which were to serve as prototypes were developed in a limited number of locations – initially at the Centre for Comprehensive Services in Carbondale, Illinois, followed by the Transitional Living Centre of Casa Colina Hospital in Pomona, California, and then the Centre for Neuroskills in Bakersfield, California.

Today, the concept of transitional living has broadened in its scope to include a wide variety of post-acute residential options. From the late 1970s when 3-4 programmes were available in the USA, there are now 47 (Fryer and Joyce, 1986).

9.1 TRANSITIONAL LIVING CENTRES

There are many interpretations on the implementation of transitional living models, grown out of a perceived need for alternatives to acute rehabilitation care. The geographical location, size and design of the physical plant are important factors to consider in order to deal best with the needs of the clients. Also important is the ability to focus assessment on observed functional abilities in everyday life and subsequently plan treatment approaches to address those needs. Even more important is understanding the concept of the transitional living model. Wood (1987a) offers a view of the role and function of transitional living by describing brain injury rehabilitation as a means of helping individuals learn strategies that increase this level of independence, improving their chances of survival in the community and increasing the probability of obtaining employment.

In order to achieve these goals, a comprehensive programme of rehabilitation must be offered which includes the range of traditional therapies but applies them in a 'social', as opposed to a 'medical' setting. This approach provides an opportunity for treatment to be directed towards goals of community living, rather than some of the more artificial clinical objectives that have prevailed in other rehabilitation models and which sometime fail to translate clinical progress into community independence.

Arguments have been offered for taking rehabilitation out of the hospital and into the community (see Chapters 4 and 5). One reason for this is that hospitals are for 'sick people' and the role of nurses and other clinical staff is to care for them. This contradicts the philosophy of rehabilitation which is based on the premise that the individuals have to learn to look after themselves.

The transitional living model removes these basic obstacles to rehabilitation. Based around a free-standing unit in the community, it tries to create a domestic and social atmosphere, whilst still maintaining a highly structured and supervised environment. The staff are trained for, and are alert to, medical complications that may arise, although the medical aspects of treatment receive a relatively low profile. For example, while medications are closely monitored by a qualified nurse to ensure medical treatment needs are fulfilled, the residents (as opposed to patients) of the programme are taught to manage their own medication, if possible.

Priority is given to the functional and social skills that an individual will need in order to successfully re-integrate into the community. Training aims to help the person acquire the maximum level of independence possible within the constraints imposed by their disability. This may include advanced mobility techniques to overcome the various obstacles one might encounter in the community. Cognitive aspects of rehabilitation also emphasize functional skills for community living: money management and the ability to budget, planning a menu and organizing a meal, for example. Above all else, the resident has the opportunity to practice the skills where it matters – in the community. There are considerable differences in being able to walk in the safety of a hospital clinic compared to a busy street or supermarket. Similarly, a person practising money management in a speech pathologist's quiet office experiences far fewer distractions than he or she would at the bank clerk's desk or the supermarket checkout.

It is the opportunity to generalize the skills learned in therapy into the real world that characterizes the advantages of a transitional living model. Although not appropriate or necessary for all brain injury survivors, it does offer an ideal training ground for the more severe and socially inappropriate individuals who, without this type of opportunity, may be forced to remain more dependent as time passes.

Traditionally the clientele of transitional living programmes were predominantly individuals who were aiming for independent living in the community. With the changing demographics of the head-injured population, this is increasingly not the sole function of a transitional living programme. Thus, a comprehensive, integrated model which deals with the diverse needs of the head-injured is now required.

The transitional living model must see itself as a vehicle for moving a patient along the path of recovery, taking into consideration the multitude of needs a person presents. Early assessment of neurological deficits, physical limitations, medical issues and psychosocial considerations of the patient are necessary to dictate the direction that treatment must follow, as well as acting as a predictor of eventual outcome. Early assessment also highlights potential problem areas and barriers which must be overcome in order for the patient to fulfil his/her rehabilitative potential.

A broad spectrum of services needs to be inherent within the programme so that the treatment plan can take account of the needs established by the assessment. The capability to provide all clinical interventions must exist together with provision of interventions for ameliorating attention, orientation and concentration deficits, memory difficulties, physical limitations and behavioural problems. The ability to deal with each obstacle in an organized manner is highly desirable.

For example, a patient whose primary physical limitation is the inability to walk but who also presents with a severe attentional deficit, is going to achieve little progress in physical therapy, regardless of the intensity or frequency of treatment unless the attentional deficit is addressed simultaneously by the rehabilitation specialists on the team. In this example, the therapists are addressing more than would be traditionally expected of them. They are able to facilitate progress in both areas by the simultaneous treatment of both deficits. Thus, a programme needs to be structured so that the treatment team is involved in reciprocal treatment approaches to address multiple patient's needs. Regardless of the deficits, the treatment focus must be on functional goals which have a practical application for the individual's long-term future.

The environment of a transitional living programme lends itself naturally to the training of functional skills because, in most cases, it closely resembles the environment in which the person will be using those skills. It is incumbent upon the programme, therefore to use the environment to its full potential. To this end the therapy day should primarily take place within the community and residential environment. Upper extremity range of motion, for example, can be achieved through hanging laundry on a clothes line as opposed to an unrelated range of motion exercises in a clinic. On a more advanced level, it is much more practical to teach budgeting skills in a bank or supermarket with all the potential complications of that situation than attempting to train the same skill in an unrelated setting. One cannot assume, however, that the skill will automatically generalize to the community. Repetition of skills training in the functional settings available to a transitional living programme, enhances the generalization of these behaviours.

The treatment team

The clinical treatment team of a transitional living centre does not differ a great deal from that present in a traditional rehabilitation setting. The team consists of speech pathologists, occupational therapists, recreational therapists, psychologists, physical therapists, a physician, licensed nursing personnel, a vocational specialist and a group of specially trained rehabilitation assistants and case managers. This may seem like a heavy load of professional personnel for a transitional programme; yet there is a major distinction between this type of rehabilitation programme and a residential living programme. Traditionally, residential living programmes have provided maintenance or custodial care. The transitional programme being described in this chapter provides intensive restorative rehabilitation with social, cognitive, behavioural, vocational and physical goals, requiring relevant rehabilitation specialists.

These professionals must act in concert, as an interdisciplinary team in order to maximize their effectiveness. There has been a great deal written about the functioning of an interdisciplinary team and the positive impact this method of organizing staff energy can have on a treatment plan. It is especially true in the treatment of head injuries. Each member of the treatment team will bring specialized skills to the case. The physical therapist may primarily focus on mobility skills, the occupational therapist on functional activities of daily living and the psychologist on issues of behaviour and adjustment. However, these therapists and the rest of the team also have an additional responsibility to the patient's long-term goal and the treatment plan as a whole. Under these circumstances, each member of the treatment team shares the responsibility of identifying treatment needs and participating in remediating problems. An example may help clarify this point.

Case example

A 20 year old man (Mike) has suffered a head injury which has left him with residual deficits including: reduced attention span, increased distractability, uninhibited and impulsive behaviour. His physical status is good yet he requires supervision for all activities of daily living because he lacks the organizational abilities and safety judgement upon which community independence largely depends. The targets of the treatment team included independent ADL (activities of daily living) skills, supervised living in a hostel and some form of sheltered employment. At this time his primary rehabilitation issues are:

1. Distractability combined with an inability to maintain attention to task; this deficit results in his spending up to 2 hours completing a morning hygiene programme, because he is distracted by the activities of other people who share the same living environment.
2. Poor social presentation; approaches others by hugging and constant handshaking.
3. Intermittent fidgeting (scratching, rubbing body parts etc.).

It is important to note that the entire therapy team have adapted their treatment techniques in order to apply them to Mike's rehabilitation goals. One can assume that the therapists are choosing which tasks to use as therapeutic opportunities based on the goals that are present and that the structure of the programme allows for specific individuals to be responsible for certain aspects of the day. These three rehabilitation issues become the focus of his treatment plan at this time and all the therapists have these items as the primary team goals. The importance of this approach is clear; the treatment team needs to deal with these basic skills first in order to establish a base of abilities that can be built upon. By sequentially providing Mike's treatment services as an interdisciplinary unit, the therapy team does not waste time or resources and can get optimal responses from Mike. An example of Mike's therapy day is as follows:

Time of day   *7-8 a.m.*

Task   *Rise/grooming and hygiene*

Therapeutic intervention.   *Mike has 1:1 staff to cue simple steps of his morning programme. Included in such steps are:*

'Mike, get up; get your robe; grab your towel, grooming kit' etc. *For every four cues that are carried out within 30 seconds of the cue being given, Mike is rewarded with extra praise. If the tasks are not carried out, the cue is repeated until the tasks are completed. At the end of the entire task, feedback is given to Mike on how many extra cues he required and this is recorded on his wall chart.*

Time of day   *8-8.30 a.m.*

Task   *Prepare/eat breakfast*

Therapeutic intervention.   *Mike is cued to attend to the task of preparing and eating breakfast by using a simple phrase 'look at . . .' when assisting him with attending to the task. He has 30 minutes to complete eating breakfast, receiving constant verbal interaction as he attends to the task.*

Time of day   *9-9.30 a.m.*

Task   *Clean-up*

Therapeutic intervention   *Again, the cue of 'look at . . .' is used along with simple instructions as the task is completed.*

Time of day   *9.30-10 a.m.*

Task   *Orientation/planning*

Therapeutic intervention   *Mike spends the next part of the morning planning for the day. He is asked to sit in a straight backed chair with his schedule book. He is to copy his daily schedule from the master sheet. A member of staff is in the room for questions.*

Time of day *10-11 a.m.*

Task *Social skills*

Therapeutic intervention. *Mike is cued by one of the staff to determine the activities of the next day (which, in this example, is social skills). Social skills focuses on the correct social approach. Today the task involves going to the local convenience store to buy a magazine. As part of social skills, there is a role play of what is going to happen and some examples of the correct way to deal with this social situation. Basic issues are proper facial expressions, keeping his hands in his pockets, ask only for what he needs, what kind of change to expect etc. Once this has been accomplished, the group is taken to the store to complete the task. Mike is shadowed by the staff who only intervene if he has difficulty.*

Time of day *11-11.30 a.m.*

Task *Break*

Therapeutic intervention. *Mike has the opportunity to spend 30 minutes at the activity of his choice. The activities available to him are based on his level of participation during the previous 3 hours.*

Time of day *11.30-12.30 p.m.*

Task *Disability adjustment group*

Therapeutic intervention. *Mike is involved with a number of others who are at approximately the same stage in their recovery. The focus of the group is identification of things that have changed since their head injuries. In addition to providing input to the group, Mike is cued to attend to the task. The group is run by the psychologist and rehabilitation aides.*

The rest of the day adopts a similar pattern. The therapists are using the different tasks and groups as tools to get the therapy goals accomplished. For example, in the afternoon the speech pathologist might spend time with Mike following up the shopping trip, working on additional skills and social presentation.

In the example above all of the clinical therapists use the daily tasks and training groups as therapeutic tools to focus on the goals of treatment. In addition, the therapists, by working in this type of environment, can act as teachers to each other so that a speech pathologist can provide some input to physical issues and a physical therapist can impact positively on the cognitive issues. This type of an approach within a transitional living programme can have a tremendous effect on the implementation of the interdisciplinary team's programme.

One final note: Mike's therapy was geared towards someone who had mastered certain basic skills. In the case of a lower functioning person, it may be necessary to provide more basic interventions which require a separate room, more equipment etc. This situation should not change the basic interdisciplinary service delivery model but the individual needs of the person should be taken into account when planning treatment.

9.2 TREATMENT PLANNING

The planning for interdisciplinary treatment cannot be accomplished in a vacuum. Two very important components must be in place for the treatment team to function effectively. The therapists are significantly involved in the setting of treatment priorities and the ongoing clinical decision making, making it necessary for someone to have overall coordination and control of the process. This is the responsibility of the clinical coordinator. The coordinator maintains a broad perspective of the case as well as working with the therapists to identify the treatment issues, set priorities and generally be responsible for moving the rehabilitation process along. The role of the clinical coordinator will be discussed in greater detail later in this chapter.

The second component essential to an effective treatment team is the completion of functional assessments. Every member of the team completes and assesses the individual's deficits, strengths and therapy needs. Within the structure of a post-acute rehabilitation programme the neuropsychological assessment can prove to be especially significant, if completed and utilized properly. Wood (1987b) argues that the neuropsychological assessment is a crucial element of effective planning. However, he goes on to assert that many neuropsychological tests do not provide the input necessary to understand the brain-behaviour relationships at a sufficient level to promote the development of functional treatment plans (see Chapter 12 for a similar view). Within a transitional living programme a neuropsychological assessment must not only describe the type and degree of demand but pinpoint the specific approaches which can most effectively remediate the problem. Armed with a neuropsychological assessment of this nature the coordinator and the treatment team have a very clear and concise guide to planning a treatment programme.

Behavioural approaches

The value of a behavioural approach in a rehabilitation programme is that it offers a structured and systematic method through which specific functional skills and cognitive deficits can be measured (Wood, 1987a). This allows comparisons of a patient's performance to be monitored over time and can improve the efficiency of learning and subsequently the outcome of rehabilitation training. Additionally, a properly implemented behavioural approach enables the treatment team to address the problematic behaviours which often accompany head injury, and to focus on specific target behaviours, thereby allowing more effective use of time and effort.

The behavioural approach in a transitional living programme encompasses two distinct components. The first acknowledges that rehabilitation requires active participation from the patient. To put it plainly, you cannot *do* rehabilitation *to* someone; one must gain the *cooperation* of the patient. There must be a feedback system to the patient within a framework of unconditional positive regard and encouragement which consistently reinforces the participation of a patient in treatment. This system may be as simple as verbal praise when desired behaviour occurs, or may utilize a token or point system as a method of providing reinforcement for achieved goals in the therapy programme.

The second component identifies behaviours, which by their presence or absence interfere with effective treatment. Subsequently, specific behaviour interventions can be developed to deal with these issues.

Case example

Problem *T.M. is an individual whose access to therapies and daily activities is hampered by frustration-based aggressive behaviour. She is unable to maintain control over her physically aggressive outbursts and finds it especially difficult to do this when asked to complete a demanding task.*

Programme *Whenever physical aggression occurred, T.M. was removed from the treatment setting and placed in a situation where she could obtain no positive reinforcement for a period of five minutes (a process of time-out). Alternatively, whenever T.M. was cooperating with the scheduled activity, she was consistently praised (social reinforcement) and given opportunities to receive more tangible rewards for her efforts and behaviour. Figure 9.1 describes her progress during this attempt at 'differential reinforcement of other behaviour' (DRO).*

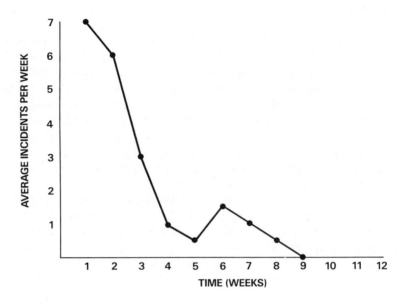

Figure 9.1 T.M.: management of aggression.

The significance of this type of treatment programme for difficult and threatening behaviour, is that it was carried out in a 'domestic setting', an ordinary home environment rather than a psychiatric unit or some other clinical setting. The latter may have made the treatment easier to administer, but the generalization of the more controlled behaviour would have been more difficult to achieve.

Cognitive approaches

Miller (1984) suggests that the purpose of cognitive rehabilitation is to assist the individual in functioning as well as possible, despite the existing handicaps. The emphasis in rehabilitation must be to develop relevant methods for training the brain-injured in the re-acquisition of skills necessary for activities of daily living. In a transitional living context there is the additional need to re-establish cognitive skills in a way which will allow these functional skills to be utilized in a variety of settings.

Initially, the aim is to identify the nature of the deficits which are impeding a particular daily living skill. It is then necessary to discover the best method by which an individual can learn a strategy to complete the skill, either through a process of 'compensation' or by a process of 'shaping' new skills. Miller describes this broad approach to cognitive training as **amelioration**. This approach accepts that there will be a certain degree of permanent deficit. For example, a person with a memory problem has a reduced ability to remember new information. Specific and controlled cognitive retraining has demonstrated improvement in some measures of memory as compared to a baseline (Wilson, 1987). However, it has not been established that this improvement can be generalized to a variety of settings, and increasing scepticism is being expressed about the clinical utility of specific memory training techniques (see Schacter et al., 1985; Wood, 1986). The essential problem with memory training is that specific strategies can be learned but, as Wood (1987b) asserts, these strategies are not necessarily successfully applied to day-to-day behaviours. Therefore, the goal of cognitive rehabilitation in a transitional living context is to select targets which are perceived to have the greatest impact on the resident's daily functioning. It must provide an opportunity for the resident to practice techniques and strategies in a real-life setting that will lead to an amelioration of deficits and help the individual gain confidence in applying a functional or social skill in a way which produces rewarding consequences. In this respect, the aim of cognitive rehabilitation is to reduce social handicap imposed by a cognitive deficit, not to reduce the deficit itself – a goal which may be impossible in the circumstances of the brain injury.

9.3 VOCATIONAL ISSUES

Of critical importance in the delivery of post-acute rehabilitation services is the ability to establish positive long-term outcomes. Many areas of a person's life must come together in order to achieve the long-term success that everyone strives for. Included in these areas are an intact support system, healthy leisure opportunities and, in most cases, participation in meaningful work-related activities. The latter issue, work, takes on a special significance when one considers the age and work potential of the great majority of the head-injured. Injuries as a whole account for more loss of pre-accident pursuits than heart disease and stroke combined. Given that the National Head Injury Foundation (1980) estimates conservatively that there are 75 000 new incidences of head injury each year, it becomes a top priority within a transitional living programme to make provision for the vocational rehabilitation of clients. It is necessary to introduce training early on in the course of treatment and integrate that training as a primary element of rehabilitation – not as an afterthought, as seems to be the case in many rehabilitation programmes.

The vocational rehabilitation approach used in a transitional living programme consists of five major phases: assessment, treatment, work administration, vocational training and transitional employment. The following provides a brief overview of each of these phases and their contribution to the eventual outcome.

Assessment phase

The assessment phase is designed to identify and provide training for the development of basic cognitive, physical and behavioural skills needed within a vocational environment. It is provided to those residents who have been identified as potential candidates for return to some level of work. The term 'work' in this context is defined as an activity directed towards some meaningful purpose, be it a therapeutic activity, simulated work, supported employment, education activity or competitive employment. An accurate assessment can facilitate the transition of a person's vocational potential through the subsequent phases by establishing a strong foundation of skills. The sequence of events which can occur within this prevocational phase include:

Overview assessment.   This involves the completion of a preliminary assessment by the treatment team and the vocational specialist. The emphasis is on identifying existing deficits which will impact on the individual's ability for more advanced vocational training. The overview assessment needs to be completed early in the rehabilitation process so specific intervention techniques can be implemented as part of the treatment plan.

Utilization of therapeutic 'work' tasks.   It is important for the treatment team and the vocational specialist to work closely together to design simultaneous work tasks which will address the existing deficits. By utilizing the many 'work' opportunities that are available within a transitional living environment they can obtain significant feedback regarding a person's potential for further vocational training.

Contact with previous employer.   Part of the assessment phase needs to include contact with the pre-accident employer (if appropriate) to determine the feasibility of returning to that employer as well as the necessary conditions for this to happen.

Preparation for the treatment phase

As previously stated, the assessment phase is intended to set a firm foundation for further training. Areas which need to be considered for remediation within this phase include:

Cognitive.   In order to address the variety of situations a person must face, basic cognitive skills need to be established. These cognitive skills include, but are not limited to: attention, memory, organization and planning. Treatment within therapeutic work tasks may focus on the ability to do any of the following:

1. sustain and shift attention
2. concentrate in a distracting environment
3. take in new information and begin following more than one-step commands
4. organize activity
5. begin utilizing compensatory strategies

Physical.   The training in the assessment phase should focus on the physical abilities which may be needed for work. When appropriate, assistive devices or task modifications may be necessary to compensate for certain physical limitations. The following areas may be considered for treatment:

1. advanced ambulation skills
2. gross/fine motor coordination
3. capacity for exertion
4. endurance for sustained movement
5. speed and accuracy

Behavioural.   Emphasis on behavioural issues can be provided for those patients who have gained some control over their behaviour. Treatment considerations may include the following areas:

1. social skills development
2. adjustability
3. tolerance to feedback from others
4. social interaction pattern with peers and others

The treatment phase

The focus of the treatment phase is to take the information which has been generated throughout the assessment phase and add to it specifically designed systematic evaluation measures. The end result will be the development of a vocational rehabilitational plan. The main components of the treatment phase include:

Formal vocational evaluation. Within the treatment phase, a comprehensive vocational evaluation may be completed. The important factor to plan for is the specialized design of the evaluation. There are many vocational testing batteries available but these are not necessarily appropriate to the needs of a head-injured person. Added to this, much of the information needed may already have been obtained through the assessment phase. It is extremely important for the vocational specialists to design a test battery which will address the issues at hand, minimizing the redundancy of information.

Up to this point, most of the vocational plan has been implemented as part of the treatment environment within a transitional programme. As a patient reaches the next phase of vocational training, the emphasis and location of treatment changes. This is especially important in a transitional living programme where the emphasis needs to shift, from medical to social rehabilitation issues. As the priorities of treatment shift, so too must the focus of the staff providing therapy. The coordination of this shift in treatment priorities is a primary role of the clinical coordinator (sometimes referred to as a case manager).

Work assimilation. There are a variety of training foci that can be provided within the work assimilation phase, depending on the needs of the individual and the direction of the treatment plan. There are three types of approach which help the patient adapt skills and behaviours developed in earlier stages of their rehabilitation to the work setting. They can be used together or individually.

1. *Work hardening.* There will be circumstances when patients have limited physical tolerance. Work hardening focuses on physical development with tasks specific to the workplace.
2. *Work adjustment.* The emphasis of work adjustment is to maintain the previously learned behaviours in a work environment. Here the individual has the opportunity to develop comprehensive job skills. Because many head-injured individuals may have difficulty generalizing previously learned skills and strategies to new environments, this component can be especially helpful to a successful vocational outcome.
3. *Supported work.* This component trains the individual on specific work tasks within a work environment. These training experiences

may take place in job stations, in or around the transitional living programme or, in the case of higher level individuals, within designated business sites in the community. An important element of this approach is the use of job coaches to assist the patient at the work site and facilitate consistent feedback.

Vocational training.   Vocational training as a component of the vocational rehabilitation plan deals with the development of specific skills which will eventually lead to placement. An important element is 'on the job training'. Here a relationship is established with an employer, with the employer agreeing to provide on-the-job training for an individual. Usually, the employer agrees to pay a certain percentage of the wage with the expectation that, as the person develops skill and knowledge of the job, the employer's percentage grows to the point where the person holds a regular position in the company. For those individuals who reach this phase of training, a great deal of interaction and planning needs to take place between the vocational specialist and the employer, using good job analysis and clinical information as a basis for decision making.

There are a number of training opportunities that include specific skills (e.g. industrial training, clerical training, janitorial training, assembly training etc.). These alternative occupations can be effectively used as training sites that may well be turned into placement sites if appropriate. It is not clear how many of these opportunities exist or the degree to which they are appropriate for vocational training. The vocational specialist must closely scrutinize options which become available to make sure they fit the specific needs of the head-injured client and do not require cognitive, physical or social skills that are beyond the client's range of ability.

Transitional employment.   The goal of implementing a systematic training programme of this nature is for the person involved to be able to return to some form of gainful employment. However, if one looked at a head-injury population and the continuum of work activities which are available, one would see one group of individuals being inappropriate for work at any level, and another group capable of normal employment. Inevitably there is a mid-point to this continuum, represented by a host of supportive and sheltered work opportunities. Patients who are involved in a transitional living programme would span this continuum, but, even more importantly, a large percentage would be in the mid-range. This has serious implications for the transitional living programme that targets vocational outcomes as one of the patient's goals. Placement may often mean creating a work situation where the individual can best function given the limitations he/she may have. This can be with previous employers or in an entirely new setting. The important fact is that the treatment team must be creative when planning for placement alternatives and must have the capability of follow-up at the work site, on a frequent basis if necessary, in order to facilitate a good long-term outcome.

9.4 THE FAMILY AS A KEY TO TREATMENT

Needless to say, the focus of a transitional living programme is the patient. However, the patient's support system, usually the family, requires a great deal of attention as well. Within the structure of a transitional living programme several methods of intervention may be desirable, depending on a particular family's abilities and level of understanding. For example, educating the family on how to deal with long-term issues may be both helpful and necessary to achieve successful long-term results. How well this information is received by the family relies on critical variables such as the timing of introduction of the information, the amount and nature of the information and the status of the staff person relating the information. Rosenthal and Muir (1983) discuss this point when identifying the factors to consider before initiating intervention. They stress the importance of addressing needs a family may have, and go on to divide family intervention techniques into two broad categories: those conducted by rehabilitation professionals and those conducted by non-professionals (e.g. peers, families). To be effective in dealing with the myriad of family issues within post-acute services the programme needs to make provisions to provide or coordinate the delivery of a number of techniques within the following broad categories.

Family education.   Family education has received a great deal of attention over the past several years and there have been a number of good educational programmes developed. The main topics for an educational series may include cognitive deficits, behaviour management, socialization, vocational opportunities, communication etc. Family education can also have a secondary gain: peer support.

Supportive counselling.   The major goal of supportive counselling is to assist the family in the mourning process that accompanies adaptation to having a head injury survivor in their midst. In a transitional living programme this can be accomplished by the clinical psychologist, but the support that the family needs can also be offered by the other rehabilitation professionals in the team, adding to the frequency of support.

Family therapy. In their discussion of 'Methods of Family Intervention', Rosenthal and Muir (1983) describe the focus of family therapy as being the entire family unit. Because of the variety, great care should be taken prior to instituting family therapy to ensure that the patient can manage to understand the nature of the discussion, and cope with the emotional issues that emerge from that discussion, in order to participate meaningfully in the therapy process.

Specific training/participation in treatment. This involves training the family in methods of caring for a relative who is about to return home and is usually based upon a specific plan for the family to implement techniques developed in the transitional living programme. The transitional living setting is particularly appropriate for this type of training because the environment is often much like the home setting. For those families who will continue to provide long-term support for the patient, this aspect of training can be most productive in increasing their understanding of the problems they are likely to encounter and how to deal with them. Often training alone is not enough, however, and the family member may gain more skill and insight by participating in the actual treatment proces. In this kind of treatment setting there are many opportunities in which a family member can participate. Additionally, this approach can be used to facilitate the families' support of the treatment plan.

Trial visits to the family home. Therapeutic visits can be especially useful in determining the feasibility of the family home as a discharge site. In addition to giving the patient and the family the chance to have some time in the home away from the treatment setting, this approach offers a unique opportunity to see the family as a unit. It is advisable to provide the patient and the family with specific assignments to obtain feedback on the family's abilities and desire to deal with the family member in the home.

Family (peer) support groups. Often, a family will need the empathy and advice of someone who has gone through a similar experience. Thus, support groups assembled from families who have experience or who are experiencing such a treatment process are of tremendous value. The treatment team should provide the family with the resource information about local community support groups.

While the family of a head-injured person can often be central to the rehabilitation process, the patient must remain the main focus of attention. This is not a simple concept that is managed by treatment plans alone; rather, it is a question of philosophy and attitudes. It requires an awareness that in order to implement successfully a flexible and sophisticated therapy programme, the training is and supervision should be applied to a patient and family with unconditional positive regard. This does not mean that the patient is always correct or that the therapists should not provide certain services because that patient does not want them. It means however that the patient's needs should always be considered first. This concept is especially significant in a transitional living programme where there are a number of staff providing supervision on a 24-hour basis. Conflicts are almost certain to arise and an approach that does not include positive regard as a key point can have deleterious effects on the patient's participation in the programme as well as the patient/staff relationship, and hence on the ability to provide a successful rehabilitation service.

Additionally, the programme must consider the patient's rights. This goes beyond the obvious rights which deal with privacy, food and sleeping quarters. As Keister (1985) described in his discussion on 'patient empowerment', one focus of the rehabilitation programme is to 'restore all the power of self-direction, choice and self-initiation as quickly as the patient can safely exercise these powers'. This concept, carefully implemented, can have enormous impact and has significant implications for a transitional living programme. It is clearly the goal of treatment to ease people out of the 'programme' into the mainstream of society, if at all possible. Patient empowerment is not extrinsic to this process, rather it is the essence of it. Too often we tend to make patients too dependent on a therapy programme, demanding compliance in every detail of daily living. A transitional living approach which deals with the issue of greater independence for the patient by planning for increasing levels of self-direction will have taken a major step towards making this goal a reality.

9.5 CLINICAL TREATMENT PLANNING AND STAFF COMMUNICATION

An effective framework for treatment planning, decision-making and communication is required in order that the different elements of rehabilitation can be properly implemented. Earlier, we spoke of clinical coordination (or case management) as one of the keys for effective treatment planning. This approach, utilizing systematic mechanisms for planning and 'single point' accountability for monitoring goals has proved to be very effective in keeping the rehabilitation programme on track, and controlling the treatment process by maintaining a broad view of rehabilitation goals in relation to the established 'outcome goal' (see Chapter 6). Only by having a clear perspective on different treatment goals can effective long-term clinical management take place.

The case management system which we advocate in a transitional living programme has one or more individuals, depending on the programme's census, acting as programme case managers. These individuals are essentially the clinical team leaders. They attend and coordinate all of the team meetings related to the treatment planning for a patient, keep track of all of the issues which may impact on the case, and continually direct the team to the primary rehabilitation issues. This position demands an understanding of the skills of all the members of the clinical team in order to direct effective clinical decisions.

For the programme case managers to be effective, the system of treatment planning and service delivery must be interdisciplinary. This allows the programme case manager to work with the team to set functional goals which relate to a patient's practical needs. Too often, rehabilitation programmes focus on the contribution of individual disciplines to the patient's treatment rather than maintaining a more holistic approach to rehabilitation. A well implemented interdisciplinary approach, coordinated by a case manager, can transcend the traditional rehabilitation schemes by facilitating optimal management and outcome.

Two components which are essential to this process are the case conference and the treatment planning meetings. The case conference can be the main occasion for evaluating results, and discussing a resident's long-term plans. An interdisciplinary framework allows the case manager and the team to work together to determine primary areas of treatment. The case conference format also allows good communication between the team members so that they all approach the plan with the same basic knowledge. Additionally, the case conference can be used as a mechanism for formal presentation of progress to the family (and insurance agent, if appropriate) including information on functional status, progress and long-term plans.

Very often, case conferences do not allow sufficient time to discuss and plan specific intervention measures which need to be implemented by the interdisciplinary team. Alternatively, treatment planning meetings allow specific treatment methods to be determined and integrated into the general programme of therapy. Most of the cases in a transitional living programme are very complex. It is therefore necessary to deal with a multitude of long-term cognitive, behavioural and social problems that have implications for community re-entry. An integrated treatment plan can keep each of these problems areas in focus, allowing staff to maintain a balance between immediate treatment needs and long-term objectives that will improve the patients' quality of life and increase the reliability of their remaining as independent members of the community.

9.6 SUMMARY

A catastrophic event such as a head injury puts into motion a series of medical interventions which are intended to save the individual's life and to rehabilitate the person as closely as possible to their premorbid self. As recent studies have demonstrated (Brooks et al., 1986; Livingston et al., 1985; Brooks and McKinlay, 1983), once a head-injured person and his or her family have passed the stage of medical stability, the ongoing issues of psychosocial development and community reintegration may continue to be a struggle. In the past, head-injured individuals were relegated to an inadequate system of care. Not until the late 1970s did more specialized programmes designed to address the long-term needs begin to develop. Today, a relatively large number of transitional living programmes are in existence with more being developed every year. Recent statistics indicate that, unfortunately, the demand for these types of programmes continues to exceed the supply.

For a transitional living programme to meet this growing demand, it must be capable of addressing a wide variety of patient needs in a comprehensive and coordinated manner. The programme must operate in a comprehensive and coordinated manner, and must be able to assess and develop functional skills which will facilitate greater independence in daily living. Short-term outcome studies are just beginning to demonstrate the efficacy of transitional living programmes and their place in the rehabilitation continuum. Undoubtedly, the analysis of these studies and the ones that follow will contribute to the emerging technology and allow further refinement of the services that are provided.

REFERENCES

Brooks, D.N. and McKinlay, W.W. (1983) Personality and Behavioural Changes After Severe Head Injury: A Relatives View. *J. Neurol. Neurosurg. Psychiat.*, **46**, 336–44.

Brooks, D.N. *et al.* (1986) Five Year Outcome of Severe Blunt Head Injury: A Relatives View. *J. Neurol. Neurosurg. Psychiat.*, **49**, 764–70.

Fryer, J. and Joyce, D. (1986) Survey of Post-Acute Rehabilitation Programmes. Results of survey presented at the Seventh Annual Braintree Conference, October 8, Braintree, MA.

Keister, M.E. (1985) *Liberty and the Pursuit of Happiness After Brain Damage: Patient Choice in Rehabilitation.* Presented at the American Congress of Rehabilitation Medicine, Kansas City, MO, September 30.

Livingston, M.G., Brooks, D.N. and Bond, M.R. (1985) Patient Outcome in Year Following Severe Head Injury and Relatives Psychiatric and Social Functioning. *J. Neurol. Neurosurg. Psychiat.*, **48**, 876–81.

Miller, E. (1984) *Recovery and Management of Neuropsychological Impairments*, John Wiley, New York.

National Head Injury Foundation Publication (1980), Framingham, MA.

Rosenthal, M. and Muir, C., (1983) Methods of Family Intervention, in *Rehabilitation of the Head Injured Adult* (M. Rosenthal *et al.*, eds), F.A. Davies Co., Philadelphia, pp. 407–16.

Schacter, D.L., Rich, S.A. and Stampp, M.S. (1985) Remediation of Memory Disorders: Experimental Evaluation of the Spaced-retrieval Technique. *J. Clin. Exp. Neuropsych.*, **7**, 79–96.

Wilson, B.A. (1987) *Rehabilitation of Memory*, Guilford Press, New York.

Wood, R.Ll. (1986) Rehabilitation of Patients with Disorders of Attention. *J. Head Traum Rehab.*, **1** (3), 43–53.

Wood, R.Ll. (1987a) *Brain Injury Rehabilitation: A Neurobehavioural Approach*, Croom Helm, London; Aspen Publishers, Rockville, MD.

Wood, R.L. (1987b) Neuropsychological Assessment in Brain Injury Rehabilitation, in *Advances in Clinical Rehabilitation* (M.G. Eisenburg and R.C. Grzesiak, eds), Springer, New York.

Young, J.S., *et al.* (1982) *Report on Spinal Cord Injury Statistics: Experience of the Regional Spinal Cord Injury Systems*, Good Samaritan Medical Centre, Phoenix, AZ.

10 Risk-benefit considerations in drug treatment

Peter Eames

Pharmacology is the scientific study of the effects of drugs on biological systems, and therapeutics is the study of the practical use of drugs in the treatment of human illness. Clearly there is a strong connection between them, but there are also important but often hidden differences between the mental attitudes which govern their use. Ideally, every act of prescription should be based on the consideration of pharmacological knowledge. Unfortunately, pharmacology is generally taught at a time, during preclinical studies, when actual patients and the drama of practical medicine are but a glint in the eye of the student; thus it tends rather to be feared as a 'dry' subject. Therapeutics, on the other hand, is taught alongside the other aspects of clinical medicine, in an automatically integrated way, and is therefore much more exciting and immediate. Moreover, rather a large proportion of available treatments have an empirical basis – which is a more impressive way of saying that we do not know how or why they work. Understandably, therefore, doctors often react to a medical condition by thinking automatically of the 'appropriate' drug treatment, in a way which bypasses thinking about pharmacology. This almost subliminal sort of training would work very well, but for the fact that most drugs have more than the one pharmacological action which is 'appropriate' to any particular condition.

A common example of this problem is that many doctors, when presented with a complaint of dizziness and vomiting react almost automatically with prochlorperazine (Stemetil, Compazine), yet relatively few are aware that this drug is a phenothiazine, effective in the treatment of schizophrenia, and can therefore provoke acute dystonia and other extrapyramidal disorders. It is often automatically prescribed as 'one tablet three times a day', often in ignorance of the fact that it is available in tablets of either 5 mg or 25 mg. (I once met with a mini-epidemic of acute dystonia – misdiagnosed inevitably as hysteria – caused by a combination of this method of prescribing with the fact that the pharmacy had acquired a large supply of 25 mg tablets by mistake!)

Pharmacological effects other than the desired one are often referred to as 'side-effects'. This is a pity, because it encourages the idea that they are somehow incidental. They are in fact every bit as much *direct* effects of the drug as is the wanted one, and it is a salutory practice to get into the habit of calling them 'unwanted effects'. An example may help to underline this point. One drug manufacturer markets orphenadrine hydrochloride as a muscle-relaxant, without mentioning in the data sheet that it is an anticholinergic agent useful in the treatment of Parkinsonian disorders. A different company markets the same drug as an anti-Parkinsonian agent, without mentioning that it is a muscle-relaxant. Which is the side-effect here?

It is obvious that the best way to use drug treatments in any condition is to consider not only how to achieve the desired effect, but also the possible consequences of other pharmacological effects of drugs which may achieve this. In the management of head injury, however, whether in the acute stage or during rehabilitation and resettlement, there are reasons for being particularly cautious whenever a drug treatment is being considered. The most pressing reason is that head injury of any severity always produces deficits of arousal, drive and attention, and many drugs (whether aimed at brain functions or not) have a tendency to sedate, and thus to exacerbate these neuropsychological deficits. Of almost equal importance is the fact that many drugs are epileptogenic, and the development of post-traumatic epilepsy has such profoundly deleterious effects on the long-term outcome after head injury (see Chapter 11) that every effort should be made to avoid encouraging it. Also very significant is that a number of drugs, especially psychoactive ones, have been shown to reduce the brain's potential for recovery of function through mechanisms of plasticity (Feeney et al., 1982), and should therefore be avoided whenever possible. Finally, it is common experience that drugs which affect brain function may have more potent effects on the damaged brain than on the intact brain.

This chapter explores these themes, describing the safest options and the greatest risks, and suggests that the notion of balancing risks against possible benefits should become a routine part of the process of drug prescribing in the management of those who have suffered head injury. Drug treatments are considered under the headings of those used to try to reverse specific effects of injury, those aimed at complications, those used to treat intercurrent illnesses, and those used to treat intercurrent symptoms. A major theme is the avoidance of iatrogenic disorders.

10.1 TREATMENT OF DEFICITS DUE TO PRIMARY INJURY

In practice, there are as yet very few such treatments available. However, those which may be tried do not carry any great risks, and in most cases the worst that can happen is to achieve no improvement. In general, therefore, drugs in this category are often 'worth a try', since even doubt about their potential effectiveness does not outweigh their safety – basically, there is nothing to lose.

Hormones

When there is reason to think that there may have been damage to hypothalamic sources of pituitary hormones, these may be measured in the blood. If there is evidence of deficiency, replacement therapy needs to be given (for example, in the case of thyroxine), or at least considered (e.g. testosterone). In the latter case it should be remembered that male hormones are associated with aggressiveness in the normal state, and if there are already problems in this direction, they may be exacerbated (although this does not by any means necessarily occur). The restoration of normal sexual drive may be of little benefit if it is accompanied by abnormal aggressiveness, and indeed the latter may lead to dangerous or even criminal behaviour. It is important, therefore, to attempt such treatment with oral preparations in the first place, rather than with the much longer acting depot injections whose actions are not readily reversed. It is wise to undertake a trial of this sort in a setting where an increase in aggression can be easily managed, for example, a rehabilitation unit organized on behavioural lines. (In view of some of the evidence from sex hormone replacement therapy in other conditions in the female, it is possible that small doses of testosterone may be helpful in the treatment of sexual unresponsiveness following recovery from head injury.)

An important hormone subgroup is the peptide hormones. Of particular interest are vasopressin and its analogues, because there is some evidence, although by no means fully confirmed, that they may improve attention and memory (Cope, 1986). To a large extent, studies using lysine-vasopressin (LVP) by intranasal nebulized spray (Syntopressin) have shown positive results, whilst those using arginine-vasopressin (DDAVP and DGAVP), by any route, have not. LVP is used in very small doses, which are not associated with any unwanted effects (except very occasional local allergic reactions to the excipient), and is believed to be absorbed via the olfactory nerve perineural structures directly to the base of the brain. Peptides appear to exert modulatory rather than specific time-locked effects, and one of the more interesting observations on the claimed beneficial effects of LVP on attention and memory is that a period of a few weeks' treatment may produce improvements which persist in the absence of further treatment, as though the peptide had in some way reset mechanisms which then continue to function at the new level. Thyrotropin releasing hormone (TRH), which is reported to have had some success in the treatment of some depressive illnesses, can produce dramatic improvements in cerebellar ataxia of degenerative origin (Sobue *et al.*, 1980), and may occasionally help traumatic ataxia also, but can be given only parenterally, and so is of rather limited use. It is likely that attempts to produce changes after trauma with other peptides will be explored, since the diencephalon, so often damaged in brainstem injury, is rich in these substances. (The hypothalamus has been described as 'peptide soup'!)

Modulation of neurotransmitter actions

The classical neurotransmitters (NT) are principally acetylcholine (ACh), dopamine (DA), noradrenaline (NA), 5-hydroxytryptamine (5-HT) and gamma-aminobutyric acid (GABA). Some of them are known to be depleted in the acute stage of severe head injury, and the vicissitudes of the recovery period may make it difficult for the brain to restore their metabolism to normal functional levels. One way in which this may be helped is to provide high tissue concentrations of the NT precursor substance: even if the enzyme systems needed for the formation of the NT are defective, this will increase the rate of the chemical reaction (in keeping with the Law of Mass Action), and normal function may thus be made more possible. An obvious advantage of this approach is that it involves the use of substances which are not 'drugs', and which the normal metabolic systems are well equipped to deal with. A disadvantage, which may not be so obvious, is that it can have effect only if the neurons are intact.

The best known example of this sort of NT manipulation is the use of levodopa (L-dopa) in Parkinson's disease. Since extrapyramidal disorders of movement and will (called **abulia** by the neurological department at the Massachusetts General Hospital, see Fisher, 1983) are common after severe head injury, L-dopa may be of help, although the probability of damaged neurons makes it more likely that dopamine agonists like bromocriptine will be effective (Ross and

Stewart, 1981), since these act post-synaptically (on the next neuron down the line). The precursor L-tryptophan may boost 5-HT activity, and this can sometimes be effective in the treatment of depressive illness. 5-Hydroxytryptamine is involved in sleep mechanisms, and there are reports of the reversal of post-traumatic sleep disorders with L-tryptophan. Long before the era of modern anticonvulsant drugs, a study showed good effects in some forms of epilepsy from glutamic acid (Price et al., 1943), which is the precursor of GABA, the main inhibitory NT in most parts of the central nervous system. Acetylcholine appears to be an important excitatory NT in the brain, and is certainly involved in cognitive processes like memory and alertness, and also in cerebellar function. Its activity may be enhanced by the use of high doses of precursors: choline chloride can be used, but often seems to make people smell a bit fishy; lecithin appears to be effective without producing this inconvenience.

There is evidence that some NT precursors may only be available for conversion to the NT when they are in a particular 'pool' (Green and Grahame-Smith, 1976; Manyam, 1987), so that oral doses may not affect NT levels at all. However, the evidence of ultimate importance will be clinical, and there appear to be many studies which suggest the clinical effectiveness of tryptophan, and at least one suggesting that glutamic acid hydrochloride has an effect on GABA systems (Price et al., 1943).

An alternative way of boosting the effectiveness of NTs is to reduce the rate of their breakdown in the synaptic cleft. The classical example is the treatment of myasthenia gravis with anticholinesterase drugs, and the same drugs have been claimed to shorten coma and, more recently, post-traumatic confusion. The anticonvulsant drug sodium valproate (or valproic acid) is believed to act by inhibiting the synaptic inactivation of GABA. These substances, however, like the NT agonists (or analogues), are drugs with additional effects, and more care is needed to avoid unwanted effects.

Cerebral enhancers

Several drugs have been promoted as having rather special effects on brain function, simply enhancing neuronal efficiency, or offsetting the effects of cellular damage. The most benign are the high-potency B vitamin combinations, though there is no hard evidence that they have any real effect on recovery or function. The so-called **nootropic agents** (Giurgea, 1973), particularly piracetam, have the advantage of positive findings in both animal brain damage and some human trials (Wilsher et al., 1979), and are exceedingly safe agents. Indeed piracetam is currently *required* treatment in the acute stage of head injury in Germany, as far as insurers are concerned. So far, there seem to have been no large scale studies of its effects in head injury, however. Co-dergocrine mesylate (Hydergine) also has its adherents, and although again there is no definite evidence of benefit, it appears to produce very little in the way of unwanted effects, and no serious ones.

10.2 TREATMENT OF COMPLICATIONS OF HEAD INJURY

Agitation and other behavioural disturbances

By far the commonest post-traumatic conditions seeming to demand drug treatment are the products of early confusional states. Because agitation, aggression, wandering, and so on, appear most often in acute hospital settings, it is probably understandable that the first recourse is usually to sedatives. This is unfortunate for a number of reasons. Major tranquillizers with sedative action (e.g. chlorpromazine, thioridazine and haloperidol) are epileptogenic, and have been shown experimentally to delay and even prevent plastic mechanisms of neural recovery (Feeney *et al.*, 1982). They are also all to some extent anticholinergic, and are thus likely to interfere directly with cognitive processes – indeed, they may increase confusion caused by under-arousal. Moreover, almost all of them block some aspects of extrapyramidal motor control. Finally, they induce inert states which usually prevent active rehabilitation therapies. The latter may apply to the benzodiazepines (though often these simply fail to achieve anything at all), which also carry the risk of rebound precipitation of epilepsy, and rarely may provoke catastrophic rage reactions. Barbiturates are intensely soporific, and also interefere with recovery processes.

There are many other ways of trying to reduce confusion, amongst them careful attention to physical disorders and discomforts (like a full bladder, or constipation), manipulation of the physical environment, careful structuring of the social (interpersonal) environment, and the more sophisticated techniques of behaviour modification (Eames *et al.*, 1987). It is true that these approaches are difficult to apply in a busy mixed surgical ward, but if acute head injury management is concentrated into one area, so that such 'special' measures can become part of the local routines, and staff can gain consistent experience, they are much more effective and less damaging than most drug solutions.

If circumstances dictate that drugs must be used, then the safest choice seems to lie between meprobamate, chlormethiazole* and possibly lorazepam for oral use, and chlormethiazole*, haloperidol (or droperidol) and lorazepam if parenteral treatment is required. In any event, it is essential to use sufficiently high doses to control the situation, and to view the treatment as temporary, and for constant review – indeed, the best rule is to prescribe one dose at a time.

Where agitation is extreme, especially if it is accompanied by blindly aggressive behaviour (grabbing, swinging, scratching, biting), it is likely that damage to limbic structures is responsible, and remarkable transformations can be achieved with the use of carbamazepine. Propranolol has been reported to be very useful in agitation in the acute post-traumatic stage (Elliott, 1977), but it is essential to exclude a previous history of asthma before using this drug.

Aggressive behaviour which persists beyond the stage of post-traumatic confusion is very likely to respond well to carbamazepine. When it does not, low-dose meprobamate can be useful. In some cases lithium salts can be effective (Mattes, 1986, for review.) Moreover, there are syndromes of recurrent psychological disorder, which may involve aggressiveness and impulsivity (Bach-y-Rita et al., 1971; Elliott, 1976; Monroe, 1986), confusion, anxiety (Pond, 1957; Harper and Roth, 1962; Brodsky and Zuniga, 1978), or mixed affective symptoms (Gloor et al., 1982), which arise from lesions of the limbic structures, and are often well controlled by the same drugs, especially the anticonvulsants. The same appears to be true of some more pervasive mental changes (Bear, 1986). These clinical syndromes are not yet widely enough recognized, and often lead, therefore, to inappropriate (and often ineffective) treatment with psychotropic drugs, with all their attendant hazards for the head-injured.

Spasticity

Energetic treatment of spasticity in the early stages after severe injury is of great importance in the battle to minimize the development of contractures. The mainstay of treatment is physiotherapeutic skills. If spasticity-reducing drugs (baclofen, dantrolene sodium, diazepam) are to be used, it is logical to use them very early on, so that they can assist the efforts of the physiotherapist. However, they are all sedative to some extent, and whilst this may not matter too much during the post-traumatic confusional phase (apart from the possibility of increasing the degree of confusion), it becomes an increasingly important issue as awareness increases. It is essential, therefore, to keep the use of such drugs under regular review, and to institute trial reductions and stoppages from time to time, to ensure that the drug is still contributing helpfully.

Epilepsy

Among the most commmonly used anticonvulsant drugs, carbamazepine and derivatives of valproic acid produce the least disturbance of arousal and cognitive functions, whereas phenobarbitone, primidone, phenytoin and clonazepam have very significant deleterious effects (Thompson and Trimble, 1982; Trimble and Thompson, 1983; Troopin, 1983; Andrewes et al., 1984; Reynolds, 1985). Such studies have been carried out in groups of individuals without acquired brain injury; the universal presence of cognitive deficits after minor and severe head injuries (Rimel et al., 1981; Brooks, 1984) means that the unwanted drug effects are adding further insult to injury in these circumstances. Although these findings have been translated into standard practice in epilepsy centres, the majority of people with post-traumatic epilepsy are treated by surgeons and physicians who see relatively few of them (Gloag, 1985), and who are largely unaware of the neuropsychological research, and indeed of the evidence which shows that cognitive and psychosocial aspects are the most important in determining the outcome after head injury (Brooks, 1984). As a result, the traditional anticonvulsants are used, and indeed the commonest current prescription for this condition appears to be the combination of phenobarbitone and phenytoin, despite the generally agreed wisdom of monotherapy. Often a first step for rehabilitation physicians is to change the anticonvulsant treatment, which is usually a pleasing thing to be able to do, since it leads to a rapid improvement in alertness and cognitive functioning generally. Of course it would be more pleasing not to have had the induced deficit in the first place.

The evidence that carbamazepine has specific effects on aggressive and impulsive behaviour disorders, which are not uncommon after head injury (Mattes, 1986), and slightly fewer deleterious effects on cognition, makes this drug the more suitable for post-traumatic epilepsy, with sodium valproate being favoured when intractable unwanted effects (typically whole-body rashes or persistent neutropaenia) preclude carbamazepine.

Relatively benign though these drugs are, they do nevertheless have some minor effects on cognition, and some patients report improvements in alertness and energy when they stop taking them. This means that special care must be taken in reaching decisions about prophylactic treatment after head injury. This is an extremely difficult area, not least because there is no clear evidence to show whether prophylaxis is effective (McQueen et al., 1983). Treatment practices vary widely in drug selection, monitoring of compliance, and duration of treatment. Criteria for treatment also vary: most neurosurgeons and neurologists advise prophylaxis for those with the greatly increased risks demonstrated by Jennett (1975) and by Annegers et al. (1980) (fits in the first week after injury, depressed skull fracture, and intracranial haematoma), but they treat and follow up only a small proportion of the head-injured. It seems unlikely that firm evidence about the best use of the best drugs in the most suitable patients will come from anything short of a lengthy study of all of the head-injured in a set of large total populations with differing but carefully controlled treatment practices. Such a study seems unlikely to be made.

Migraine

There appear to be no problems specific to the head-injured from the use of ergot derivatives or from the main prophylactic treatments of migraine – propranolol, clonidine and pizotifen (though the last can be markedly sedative in some people). However, some second line drugs may cause problems: prochlorperazine and metoclopramide increase or induce extrapyramidal disorders, and are potentially epileptogenic; benzodiazepines are sedative, and exacerbate arousal and drive disorders.

Dizziness and vertigo

By far the commonest causes of dizziness after head injury, especially when the injury is of mild or moderate degree, are postural hypotension and positional vertigo. The former represents instability of brainstem-controlled vasomotor reflexes, is self-limiting, and is not susceptible to drug treatment. Positional vertigo produces feelings of dizziness when present in a mild and true vertigo when more severe, but it almost never responds to drug treatment, and nearly always improves slowly, disappearing in the great majority of sufferers within eighteen months. The management of both therefore, involves explanation and reassurance, coupled with advice about caution in changes of body position and head movements. Very often, however, prochlorperazine is offered, which has no useful effect, and introduces the risk of the various unwanted effects mentioned previously. If the physician's need to offer medication is irresistible, betahistine at least carries no significant risk.

Psychosis

The balance of evidence now suggests that major affective disorders (mania, depressive illness or bipolar disorders) can be caused by damage to the brain (Bracken, 1987, for review). The proportion of individuals suffering such illnesses after head injury who have a family history of affective disorder suggests that in some, at least, there is precipitation rather than causation of the illness. Nevertheless, standard treatments for the primary disorders have similar effectiveness in these cases. Manic illnesses often lead to behaviour which is sufficiently disturbed to demand the use of major tranquillizers, the most popular being haloperidol and pimozide. Because of the special risks of epilepsy, reduced brain recovery and raised susceptibility to extrapyramidal disorder in the head-injured, these drugs should be avoided whenever possible, but the need to control wild over-arousal may outweigh these considerations. The drug of choice, however, is undoubtedly lithium, its potential disadvantage being that it may take up to 2 weeks to exert its full effect. The same drug may be needed for prophylactic treatment, should affective illnesses be recurrent, but it should be remembered that it does induce a mild degree of cognitive disruption. Depressive illnesses, provided they have not been induced by prolonged use of major tranquillizers, will demand treatment with an antidepressant drug. Unfortunately almost all of these are epileptogenic: the only currently available one not to have been reported to provoke fits in the susceptible is viloxazine. An alternative approach is to try the effect of tryptophan (although this may take some weeks to produce an effect), or of low dose sulpiride*. It has to be recognized that both mania and depression may be fatal illnesses, and this must be weighed against the risks of unwanted effects of active treatment. When repeated episodes of affective disorder appear, there is a case for prophylactic treatment. Although lithium has long been the first choice for this purpose, more recently carbamazepine has been found to be effective (Post, 1982), and there are reasons for thinking that it may be particularly indicated when there is a history of head or other brain injury preceding the onset of the illness (Jampala and Abrams, 1983). Lithium does have some adverse effect on cognition, and this is a further reason for preferring carbamazepine.

Paranoid and other schizophreniform states may also result directly from head injury, onset being usually delayed for months or years (Lishman, 1978, for review). Again, selection of treatment is mainly a question of balancing the possible risks of treatment against those of the illness. The relatively new antipsychotic drug sulpiride* is a dopamine-blocking agent which shows some specificity for the mesolimbic system, and is therefore much less likely to induce extrapyramidal disorders. It is also apparently less epileptogenic than the standard antipsychotic drugs like the phenothiazines and butyrophenones. Clearly it has a strong claim to be the treatment of first choice in psychotic states after head injury.

Obsessive and compulsive disorders

Severe head injury often intensifies preexisting obsessional traits, not infrequently to the point of interfering with everyday activities through the time burdens imposed by the need to carry out rituals. The relationship between such states and obsessive and compulsive disorder without preceding head injury is not clear, but there is often a qualitative difference in the patients which has led to the use of the term **organic orderliness** to describe their behaviour. In primary disorders, the first choice drug treatment is clomipramine. This drug often induces initial unwanted effects which are very unpleasant, and it is, of course, potently epileptogenic. Moreover, the writer's personal experience does not include even one patient in whom it was effective. Behavioural treatments, with attempts to channel the tendency towards ritualization of tasks in helpful directions, seem to offer the best chances of success.

Extrapyramidal disorders

Whether these are a result of diencephalic or brain-stem damage, or are produced by the use of antipsychotic drugs, they are commonly treated with anticholinergic agents, typically benzhexol or orphenadrine. Once again there are problems because, as was mentioned earlier, cholinergic activity is centrally important to cognition, and these drugs interfere with it. Clearly they are to be avoided whenever possible. In drug-induced extrapyramidal disorders, if they cannot be avoided through the use of alternative treatments (for example, practical measures to reduce agitation, or sulpiride* for psychotic states), then perhaps amantadine should be preferred, since it has much less anticholinergic activity.

10.3 TREATMENT OF INCIDENTAL ILLNESS

Those who have suffered head injury are not, of course, exempt from other illnesses. Some will already have had chronic or recurrent illnesses requiring continuing treatment. Others may develop them. In addition there is the whole range of illnesses, serious and minor, which may befall any of us. The wise practice of medicine involves considering and planning treatment which takes into account not only the nature and demands of a presenting illness, but the context in which it appears. A severe head injury forms part of that context. It is simple enough to state that the guiding principle should be the need to consider carefully the potential special effects of drugs on the damaged brain. It is far more difficult to put this principle into regular practice.

It is perhaps easiest to remember the principle when the incidental condition requires treatment with drugs whose main desired effects are on the nervous system. Nevertheless, the needs of the immediate problem tend to become the focus of thinking, as the discussion above on the question of secondary psychotic states illustrated. Serious mental disorders of a primary nature carry the same potential for deflecting attention from the risks inherent in having an injured brain, yet the issues are the same, and consist both of the possible effects of appropriate drugs on the head injury problems, and of the risks of failing to treat the mental disorders adequately.

Even more problematic are illnesses whose treatment involves drugs which have actions primarily on other systems, but which nevertheless ordinarily have minor brain effects, or interact with others aimed at brain problems. For example, whilst most antibiotics present no risk to the management of head injury problems, tetracyclines are powerful inducers of hepatic enzymes which may significantly interfere with the effectiveness of anticonvulsant drugs, and erythromycin has been shown to produce potentially troublesome elevation of carbamazepine concentrations. The problem may operate in the other direction. Propranolol can have beneficial effects on explosive and confused behaviours, and is often an effective prophylactic in post-traumatic migraine. Unfortunately, it can be very dangerous to individuals who have a history of asthma, or to those who have even an occult degree of cardiac failure, or are prone to certain types of cardiac dysrhythmia.

It would be unrealistic to try to specify all of the direct and interactional pitfalls which may lurk behind the demands of the whole spectrum of medical treatments, but the watchwords 'think pharmacology' are commended as the best available protection.

10.4 TREATMENT OF INCIDENTAL SYMPTOMS

Probably the commonest use of drugs in normal practice is for the treatment of symptoms in the absence of a definite diagnosis of their cause. This is surely as reasonable a function of the physician now as it was in the days of Hippocrates. However, it presents an even greater barrier to the use of pharmacological thinking than do the situations discussed so far, despite the greater need for it. Most coughs and colds represent no more than a nuisance, yet patients (and nurses, in hospitals or residential placements) often solicit drug treatments for such symptoms. Many of the remedies readily available are mixtures, known by catchy trade names which effectively conceal possible hazards for the head-injured. Adrenergic drugs are usually included, which may exacerbate confusion and perceptual distortions, and almost all contain antihistamines which, having (like all of this group of drugs) phenothiazine-like activity, are potentially epileptogenic, and may also exacerbate extrapyramidal and arousal disorders.

Sleep disorders are easy to come up with a treatment for, but the benzodiazepines, the dominant drugs in this area, usually reduce cognitive efficiency, may provoke fits through withdrawal mechanisms, and in the early stages may possibly compromise the ceiling of later recovery. Even more hazardous is the use as hypnotics of drugs whose sedative actions are generally thought of as a nuisance, like (again) the antihistamines. Where it is clear that sleep disorder stems from persistent agitation with a definable cause, it is obviously better to aim treatment at the cause, whether by manipulation of the environmental factors, or, for example, the use of carbamazepine to reduce limbic disturbance. Where there is no such definable cause, L-tryptophan may be effective, and at least does not introduce any hazards.

Anxiety is a common symptom in any setting, and after severe head injury there are many circumstances which may provoke it, from the early organic disturbances of limbic function, through the dawning awareness of disability and frustration, to the stresses of attempting to relearn how to negotiate the physical and social challenges of the outside world. It is all too easy to succumb to the temptation to prescribe an anxiolytic drug to achieve a non-specific reduction of the anxiety: the alternative is the much more time-consuming task of analysing causes and designing environmental, behavioural, psychological or specific drug treatments. However, the many potential hazards of most anxiolytics for the head-injured person, and the fact that their effects are only symptomatic and thus often inadequate in the longer term, demand this more thoughtful approach. Of all currently available drugs with anxiolytic effects, the least harmful (except when there is a history of asthma) is propranolol, which may also confer other benefits such as a reduction of aggressive behaviour, or of episodes of migraine. In circumstances where there is the potential for learned (phobic) aspects of anxiety, it has the added advantage that it appears not to interfere with the processes of conditioned learning.

Allergic conditions are sometimes well-established illnesses (like asthma or hay fever, for example), but more often consist of rashes of doubtful origin. In both case, 'think pharmacology' remains the best guide to treatment in the head-injured. Many asthma treatments include adrenergic drugs which may tip the balance in borderline confusional states or perhaps even in epilepsy, and although there may sometimes be no way of avoiding this risk, it makes sense at least to try the effectiveness of disodium cromoglycate or of pure steroid preparations first. Similarly, if antihistamines can be avoided in the treatment of hay fever and allergic rashes, so much the better. As was mentioned above, tetracyclines may interfere with other drugs, including anticonvulsants, and this should be given careful consideration before they are used for the treatment of acne – it would be a very poor exchange to reduce an acneform rash at the cost of precipitating post-traumatic epilepsy!

10.5 CONCLUSIONS

Because of the vulnerability of the damaged brain to a wide range of unwanted effects, particularly compromise of cognition, and the risk of precipitating epilepsy, drug treatments require careful thought and great caution. The following rules need to be observed, and to avoid potential iatrogenic ravages, the doctor dealing with the head-injured should make them part of a well-practised routine.

1. When the prescription of any drug treatment is contemplated, make a careful diagnostic analysis of the problem to be treated;
2. Consider especially the possibility that drugs already being used may be responsible for the problem;
3. Consider next whether non-pharmacological alternatives for treatment are available;
4. If not, consider whether treatment is really necessary;
5. If it is, list the possible drug treatments, and examine all of their pharmacological actions, to determine the particular disadvantages they may have for the head-injured;
6. Consider potential interactions with other drugs already being used;
7. Select the least potentially harmful drug to try first.
8. Ensure that the need for treatment really does outweigh the

possible risks – not just the medical ones, but also the psychological and social risks.

9. Decide carefully whether the drug can be used on a single-dose basis, or needs to be regular and continued – preferring the former whenever possible.

10. Consider every prescription to be a trial of treatment: monitor its effectiveness, and review the prescription regularly.

* Indicates a drug not available in the USA.

REFERENCES

Andrewes, D.G., Tomlinson, L., Elwes, R.D.C. and Reynolds, E.G. (1984) The influence of carbamazepine and phenytoin on memory and other aspects of cognitive function in new referrals with epilepsy. *Acta Neurol. Scand.*, **69**, 23–30.

Annegers, J.F., Grabow, J.D., Groover, R.V. *et al.* (1980) Seizures after head trauma: a population study. *Neurology*, **30**, 683–89.

Bach-y-Rita, G., Lion, J.R., Climent, C.E. and Ervin, F.R. (1971) Episodic dyscontrol: a study of 130 violent patients. *Amer. J. Psychiat.*, **127**, 1473–78.

Brodsky, L. and Zuniga, J. (1978) *Refractory anxiety: a masked epileptiform disorder*, Paper presented to the 2nd World Congress of Biological Psychiatry, Barcelona.

Bracken, P. (1987) Mania following head injury. *Brit. J. Psychiat.*, **150**, 690–92.

Brooks, N. (1984) *Closed Head Injury: Psychological, Social and Family Issues*, Oxford University Press.

Cope, D.N. (1986) The pharmacology of memory and attention. *J. Head Trauma Rehabil.*, **1**, 66–69.

Eames, P., Haffey, W.J. and Cope, D.N. (1987) Treatment of behavioural disorders, in *Rehabilitation of the Child and Adult with Traumatic Brain Injury*, 2nd edn (M. Rosenthal, E. Griffiths, M.R. Bond and D. Miller, eds), F.A. Davis, Chicago.

Elliott, F.A. (1976) The neurology of explosive rage. *Practitioner*, **217**, 51–60.

Elliott, F.A. (1977) Propranolol for the control of belligerent behaviour following acute brain damage. *Ann. Neurol.*, **1**, 489–91.

Feeney, D.M., Gonzalez, A. and Law, W.A. (1982) Amphetamine, haloperidol and experience interact to affect rate of recovery after motor cortex injury. *Science*, **217**, 855–57.

Fisher, C.M. (1983) Abulia minor versus agitated behaviour. *Clin. Neurosurg.*, **31**, 9–31.

Guirgea, C. (1973) The 'nootropic' approach to the pharmacology of the integrative activity of the brain. *Conditional Reflex*, **8**(2), 108–15.

Gloag, D. (1985) Services for people with head injury. *Brit. Med. J.*, **291**, 557.

Gloor, P., Olivier, A., Quesney, L.F. *et al.* (1982) The role of the limbic system in experiential phenomena of temporal lobe epilepsy. *Ann. Neurol.*, **12**, 129–44.

Green, A.R. and Grahame-Smith, D.G. (1976) The effects of drugs on the processes regulating the functional activity of brain hydroxytryptamine. *Nature*, **260**, 487–91.

Harper, M. and Roth, M. (1962) Temporal lobe epilepsy and the phobic anxiety-depersonalisation syndrome. *Comprehensive Psychiatry*, **3**, 129–51; 215–26.

Jampala, V.C. and Abrams, R. (1983) Mania secondary to left and right hemisphere damage. *Amer. J. Psychiat.*, **140**, 1197–99.

Jennett, B. (1975) *Epilepsy after Non-missile Head Injuries*, 2nd edn, Heinemann, London.

Lishman, W.A. (1978) *Organic Psychiatry*, Blackwell, Oxford (Chapter 5).

McQueen, J., Blackwood, D.H.R., Harris, P., Kalbag, R.M. and Johnson, A.L. (1983) Low risk of late post-traumatic seizures following severe head injury: implications for clinical trials or prophylaxis. *J. Neurol. Neurosurg. Psychiat.*, **46**, 899–904.

Manyam, B.V. (1987) Influence of precursors on brain GABA level. *Clin. Neuropharmacol.*, **10**(1), 38–46.

Mattes, J.A. (1986) Psychopharmacology of temper outbursts. *J. Nerv. Ment. Dis.*, **174**(8), 464–70.

Monroe, R.R. (1986) Episodic behavioural disorders and limbic ictus, in *The Limbic System* (B.K. Doane and K.E. Livingston, eds), Raven Press, New York, pp. 251–66.

Pond, D.A. (1957) Psychiatric aspects of epilepsy. *J. Ind. Med. Prof.*, **3**, 1441–51.

Post, R.M. (1982) Use of the anticonvulsant carbamazepine in primary and secondary affective illness: clinical and theoretical implications. *Psychol. Med.*, **12**, 701–04.

Price, J.C., Waelsch, H. and Putnam, T.J. (1943) DL-glutamic acid hydrochloride treatment of petit mal and psychomotor seizures. *J. Amer. Med. Ass.*, **122**, 1153–56.

Reynolds, E.H. (1985) Antiepileptic drugs and psychopathology, in *The Psychopharmacology of Epilepsy* (M.R. Trimble, ed.), John Wiley, Chichester, pp. 49–63.

Rimel, R.W., Giordani, B., Barth, J.T., Boll, T.J. and Jane, J.A. (1981) Disability caused by minor head injury. *Neurosurgery*, **9**(3), 221–28.

Ross, E.D. and Stewart, R.M. (1981) Akinetic mutism from hypothalamic damage: successful treatment with dopamine agonists. *Neurology*, **31**, 1435–39.

Sobue, I., Yamamoto, H., Konagaya, M., Iida, M. and Takayanagi, T. (1980) Effect of thyrotropin-releasing hormone on ataxia of spino-cerebellar degeneration. *Lancet*, **i**, 418–19.

Thompson, P.J. and Trimble, M.R. (1982) Anticonvulsant drugs and cognitive function. *Epilepsia*, **23**, 531–44.

Trimble, M.R. and Thompson, P.J. (1983) Anticonvulsant drugs, cognitive functions, and behaviour. *Epilepsia*, **24** (Supple. 1), 555–63.

Troopin, D. (1983) Carbamazepine, in *Recent Advances in Epilepsy vol. 1* (T.A. Pedley and B.S. Meldrum, eds), Churchill Livingstone, Edinburgh.

Wilsher, C., Atkins, G. and Manfield, P. (1979) Piracetam as an aid to learning in dyslexia. *Psychopharmacology*, **65**, 107–09.

PART FOUR

Evaluation of outcome

11   Long-term follow-up

Chris Evans

The management and rehabilitation of patients with head injury has been taking place more or less unsung over most of this century; reports by Jacobson (1886), Cairns and Holbourn (1943), Russell (1964), Hooper (1966), London (1967; 1987), are just some examples of thoughtful papers which have been produced over this time. Stritch (1956; 1961) described the effects of trauma on the substance of the brain, and this was elaborated by Oppenheimer (1968). The work of the Glasgow team in categorizing outcome and the Coma Scale was written up by Jennett and Teasdale (1961). Brooks (1984) has drawn the threads of psychological rehabilitation together; and the Kemsley Unit in Northampton has shown a way to modify behaviour (Eames and Wood, 1985a,b). However, reading through earlier papers, and looking at new reports gives an overwhelming impression that workers are continually discovering the same information. This emphasizes the need to produce action instead of too many further reports. The following table summarizes some findings over the last 100 years!

Table 11.1 A century of reports on head injuries

Year	Author	Nature of injury	% of total
1886	Jacobson	Violence	18
		Falls	70
		Traffic accidents	7
		Unknown	5
1958	Hooper	Violence	16
		Falls	35
		Traffic accidents	39
		Unknown	10
1988	Evans	Violence	3
		Falls	4
		Traffic accidents	82
		Gunshot wound/bomb blast	8
		Sports	4

11.1 SIZE OF THE PROBLEM

There have been several recent papers assessing the incidence and prevalence of survivors, and discussing their problems (Wade and Langton Hewer, 1986; McLellan 1987; *Physical Disability in 1986 and Beyond*, Royal College of Physicians of London report; London, 1987).

In a health district with a population of 250 000 up to half a dozen survivors are to be expected at any one time who will remain in coma from accident until death. There will be dozens who sustain severe head injury, survive and become dependent, incapable of living by themselves or holding down employment. In studies from the UK and the Netherlands the figure given for return to work after severe head injury is only 15% (McLellan, in preparation), although it will be argued in this chapter that a major rehabilitation effort would enable many more patients to return to work. In addition there will be many hundreds each year who sustain slight head injury; and a percentage of these (the number is not yet clearly established) will have problems subsequently in employment or social adaptation which may not become apparent for some months or years.

Most patients who suffer head injury are young and may have a life expectancy of 40 or 50 years. Therefore, even at the present rates of injury and survival the already substantial number of patients in a community who have the effects of brain damage will increase steadily before an equilibrium is reached. Earlier in this book (Chapter 5) a model of community rehabilitation has been described, and in it the estranging nature of residential units was emphasized. In this chapter a model of inpatient rehabilitation is described. Lest it should be thought these views are mutually incompatible two points need making. The first is that a need for residential rehabilitation at an early stage is recognized, and the second is that Royal Air Force Chessington was from the beginning set up to be as like a 'normal' service unit as possible. So while the patterns of behaviour for the patients at Chessington might have seemed strange to a visitor, they were familiar to servicemen.

11.2 REHABILITATION IN THE ROYAL AIR FORCE

Royal Air Force Chessington, which subsequently became known as the Joint Services Medical Rehabilitation Unit (JSMRU) dealt with the sequelae from head injuries for over 30 years. Lewis (1966) reported that 'surprisingly many of those who had suffered severe head injury became fit enough to return to duty'. Knight (1972) confirmed this;

both attributed the success to a programme including adequate and specialized rehabilitation, and to the ambience of the unit. In 1972, there was a significant increase in the number of patients admitted following severe brain damage. It was believed that this was due more to modern management of the casualties, rather than an actual increase in accidents, although it also has to be said that the influx of patients who had been victims of terrorist activity in Northern Ireland did tend to attract a lot of much needed support. There was now a group who had survived severe penetrating injuries of the skull and brain, although most of the patients were servicemen injured in road traffic accidents (RTA) (Tables 11.2 and 11.3).

It became clear to the rehabilitation team that too little was known about methods of treatment or assessment; and that if progress were to be made towards better rehabilitation new, and more precise, methods of assessment and monitoring progress were essential. In addition there was a curiosity to know what was the end result of

Table 11.2 Causes of injury of patients at JSMRU (1973)

Nature of accident	Number
Road traffic	76
Gun shot, or bomb blast	8
Fall	4
Sports	3
Assault, industrial, other	3
Total	94

Table 11.3 The type of victim at JSMRU, if a road casualty (1974)

Type of victim	Number
Vehicle driver	23
Unprotected road user	20
Vehicle passenger	18
Motorcycle driver	12
Not recorded	2
Pillion passenger	1
Total	76

treatment. To do this, a comprehensive battery of assessments was devised and introduced, and later refined. These were to become the basic methods by which all such patients were examined when they were admitted to the unit. In this chapter only a brief description of these methods will be offered; further details have been published elsewhere (Evans, 1974; 1981).

After the assessments had been devised and used on a trial basis it was agreed that they should be used on a cohort of patients with brain damage in order to improve the information available for subsequent rehabilitation programmes. The first patients were admitted to the study in early 1973, and by the end of 1974 137 patients had been examined. Two years later it was made possible, by a grant from the DHSS, to repeat these examinations on all the patients who could be traced. It was felt important that the repeat examinations should be coupled with relevant outcome measures.

Phases of assessment

There are three distinct phases after head injury which need to be evaluated separately. The first is the severity of the original injury. Post-traumatic amnesia has been found to be a satisfactory measurement of this in the past, but, in the present series too many patients had been injured too severely for this to be relevant. It was, therefore, decided to use duration of unconsciousness as the measure of initial severity.

During the weeks and months after leaving hospital and coming into the JSMRU, comprehensive recordings were made of patient's abilities on admission, as well as any subsequent changes. These recordings were made using the new departmental assessments and comprised the second stage of the procedure. This allowed progress to be recorded carefully, and correlated with treatment, providing some record of the rehabilitation given (Evans, 1976). Preaccident assessments of intellectual ability were made for all the patients admitted to JSMRU but these will be mentioned in greater detail later.

Some years after discharge, a long-term review was done – the third phase. At this stage clinical assessments alone were not enough; the crucial question was whether the individual was successfully resettled back into his or her community. This was done using socially orientated outcome measures.

Definitions

Unconsciousness was taken as the time from the injury to the time when the patient could make a sensible response to questions. This had to be better than 'Yes' or 'No' but had regard to limitations placed on the patient by treatment (e.g. tracheostomy or wired jaw). **Post-traumatic amnesia** was recorded as the time from injury to the time that continuous day-to-day memory was re-established (Plum and Posner, 1972).

Social outcome categories

1. Accommodation options
   (a) Able to live in own home
   (b) Hostel accommodation without supervision
   (c) Hospital
   (d) Other long stay unit, e.g. Cheshire Home

2. Household or other aids and adaptations needed
   (a) Major – costing more than £100
   (b) Minor – costing less than £100

3. Employability
   (a) Return to same occupation as before injury
   (b) Return to equivalent occupation
   (c) Unemployed
   (d) Employed, but poorer status
   (e) In training centre
   (f) In sheltered workshop
   (g) Unemployable

4. Financial status
   The patient's income per annum after tax was recorded, and whether it came from employment (earned) or from compensation or pension (unearned).

5. Personal dependence
   (a) Total; equivalent to needing constant attention
   (b) Partial; attendance needed for some part of each day
   (c) Relative independence; no attendant required, but a major loss of job, or enforced social isolation was present
   (d) Independent. This did not imply normality. Aids or adaptations might be necessary, but not help from another person

Original management of the cohort

On transfer to the unit the initial interview was undertaken by a medical officer who performed a standard examination and took a conventional history. The design of the interview was, however, structured to some extent by using specially designed forms which prompted some important questions to be asked such as the duration of unconsciousness, the duration of post-traumatic amnesia (PTA) and hand dominance. In theory, such information should always be included in a medical examination but in practice looking back through previous surveys it had often been left unclear. In the event such prompts were found helpful but not, regrettably, infallible. The previous notes and X-rays were also culled for information. From this the admission summary was prepared.

The paramedical departments of the unit also undertook to complete their investigations of each new arrival within the first fortnight. Again these were done to a standardized questionnaire and proforma (Stichbury, 1975). The physiotherapy assessments, though detailed, were still capable of yes/no answers. Standard occupational therapy assessments were supplemented by extra tests designed to measure sensibility, discrimination of touch and manual dexterity. Since many of those passing through the unit had engineering experience a kit was designed in workshops which was to be assembled from a series of diagrams. In theory this was easy for anyone with workshop experience to complete. In practice it was not quite so easy as it looked since not only did the size of nuts and bolts vary, so did their threads and pitches. It proved a valuable screening system for identifying difficulties in skilled men who had a significant but not obvious deficit. It is now available commercially as part of COTNAB, which is the acronym for the Chessington Occupational Therapy Neurological Assessment Battery.

No clinical psychologist was available at the unit during the 1970s. Consequently assessments made by the speech therapy department were much more elaborate than usual. This was an attempt to make good the deficiency. The therapists devised high level assessments to allow deficits of memory, perception, comprehension, reading, expression, writing and personality to be measured and scored. It was possible to augment the speech therapy department's assessment with those of the education officer.

The use of qualified teachers in the management of brain damage was not common then (and not common enough now) but their work proved invaluable for treatment as well as assessment. The particular relevance for the head-injured patients was in establishing the extent of the pre-injury ability, and comparing this with deficits found after head-injury. It was soon realized that there was a unique source of information to be tapped. This was the record made on entry into the Armed Forces of each individual's recruit selection tests. These had been standardized in 1968 with comparable commercially available tests, and so allowed comparisons to be made for each serviceman with his own performance in tests completed before the injury (Vivash, 1973).

In addition, by using well-established service education methods and standard programmes much relevant material could be taught or re-taught. Since the techniques were mostly machine based it meant that patients could take their own pace through the programmes. Finally, the remedial gymnasts and the nursing staff designed and scored their assessments, and these gave a day-to-day measure of developing independence.

Day-to-day management

The basis of management of patients at Chessington was the same for patients with severe brain damage as for the other non-head-injured patients at the unit. The majority of patients who went to Chess-ington had sustained orthopaedic injury and most of their treatment was done in classes or individually by service remedial gymnasts, supplemented by individual treatment in other paramedical depart-ments. The same principle was applied to those who had suffered brain damage. However, it was often necessary that these patients be accom-modated in the wards rather than in the self-care billets servicemen are used to. Also, in the first days after admission work was done mostly on a one-to-one basis within the paramedical departments rather than in the classes run by the remedial gymnasts. In the later stages these classes filled any intervals between individual treatments.

As improvement took place the patient was included more into class and group. This pattern changed in the late 1970s when the principle of colocation ensured that there was to be transdisciplinary, as well as interdisciplinary collaboration (Stichbury et al., 1980). Having the classes in the remedial gymnasia always available meant that for those who could cope with it up to 6 hours specific treatment could be given daily.

Newly admitted brain-damaged patients got much support from other servicemen who were recovering from their head injuries and also from the servicemen who had injury other than brain damage. It should perhaps be explained here that orthopaedic patients were classified according to area of disability and extent of recovery. There would, for example, be recovering lower limb patients called 'static quads' (a group not yet weight-bearing but fit enough to do other exer-cises of the lower limb and able to develop upper limbs normally); 'early knees' were a group in which early weight-bearing flexions were permitted, and so on through intermediate and late groups – the latter being capable of tackling a full assault course prior to discharge to units where such a level of fitness was vital. It is in the nature of service humour that the group officially known as 'medicals', which included patients with severe brain damage, became known as 'static heads'. Nonetheless, this somewhat pejorative nickname did not prevent a lot of very valuable help being given by the abler and fitter members of the unit. In the light of present discussions about community versus 'institutional' rehabilitation it needs emphasizing that Chessington was a very close copy of a standard working unit of the Armed Forces and so was less likely to produce an alienation from peer groups.

Assessments were held weekly, and any change was recorded in as much detail as possible. Patients stayed at the unit from a few weeks to 2 to 3 years and wherever possible were resettled within the Armed Forces, but the same constraints apply to servicemen as to anyone else – they had to be fit to do their job within a reasonable space of time. In fact, during the final review of the figures, the duration of rehabilitation was calculated for 78 of the 94 patients (Figure 11.1).

Unfortunately not every patient had a discharge date recorded (*sic*) so the data is not complete, but it will be seen that the mode of length of stay at Chessington was 4 months. The average on these figures was 5.8 months.

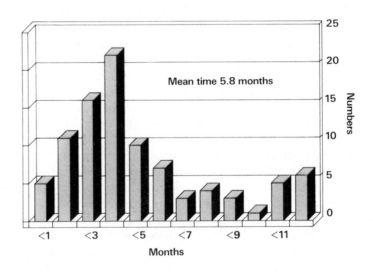

Figure 11.1 Head-injured patients: time at rehabilitation unit.

For some it was not possible for them to be re-employed in their original jobs within the Services. Under these conditions servicemen were usually offered the chance to change to a less demanding trade, and if this was not possible then they could be medically discharged from the forces. Many servicemen are on relatively short-term contracts, so that some came to the end of their contracted time before they were fit to go back to work. When this happened a resettlement programme was initiated which involved the family and the area to which the patient would be returning. This was, in any event, needed for those who were so severely brain-damaged that they would not be able to stay in the Armed Forces. This involved close liaison with civilian authorities, attempts at job resettlement, counselling, ensuring funding was appropriately established and then the care was handed over to the GPs, civilian hospitals and civilian social work services. A full formal re-examination on the scale of the entry examination took place shortly prior to discharge from the unit.

11.3 LONG-TERM FOLLOW-UP

In 1975 the DHSS agreed to fund a project for three years during which as many as possible of the original cohort of patients would be recalled and re-examined. This represented the third phase of assessment defined earlier. The work was to be done from Rivermead Rehabilitation Centre in Oxford in conjunction with JSMRU Chessington. A start was made with those who were known to still be in the Armed Forces. Two or three were brought back each fortnight to be re-examined at Chessington. This took time, but was inevitable since postings had taken some abroad and it was not considered justifiable to recall patients from abroad just for this examination. The intention was that all those followed-up should go through a medical examination using the same basic structure as on admission to JSMRU; and the same physiotherapy, occupational therapy and speech therapy assessments would also be administered.

It was clear that not all would be able to get to either Chessington or Rivermead for their reviews, so with the support of the DHSS a programme of visits was organized throughout Scotland, Wales and England to see those patients who were unable to come to Chessington or Rivermead for their re-assessments. Those who had left the Services were contacted at their last known address and where this produced no initial response they were traced through service and hospital records and through the usual NHS tracing procedure. This proved singularly effective and over the 3 years most of the patients were reviewed. Over this time over 30 000 miles were covered to find and see as many as possible of the original patients. It took 3 years to complete the collection of information. In 1982 all financial calculations were remade so that the effects of inflation on pensions and salaries in the calculations was minimized.

At the re-assessment clinics the medical examination and history was repeated, and the tests of the paramedical departments were also repeated with whatever facilities were available at the patient's home or at the local hospital (which was frequently the base for the examination). The OT tests were possible since the workshops had assembled all the tests into a portable kit (the forerunner of COTNAB).

In addition to the examinations a questionnaire was designed which was intended to illuminate changes in social habits such as hobbies, entertainment and social contacts within and outside the family. It also sought information about income; i.e. whether it was earned from a job; or unearned through pension, compensation, disability allowances or other forms of social service entitlement. There were sections asking about employment; where people lived; any complications of behaviour or any other problems which had followed the head injury, and whether any aids were needed to maintain independence. It gave an opportunity for patients and their carers to incorporate their own comments on the impact they felt that head injury had had on their subsequent life.

At the completion of the examinations, questionnaire and review of original assessment much detail concerning the accident and its immediate management had been recorded and incorporated onto summary charts together with the time of unconsciousness and PTA. These charts also displayed information about pre-injury personality and intellectual ability. The repeat examinations clarified any points of doubt in the history since relatives at this stage could supplement information and gave an extremely detailed picture of the quality of survival after brain damage. During the analysis it was hoped that clinical findings, previous employment, education and any associated injuries could be related to the final outcome measures. In the event there seemed to be close, if commonsense relationships between the outcome measures, the most telling being employability. In this chapter only scant attention will be paid to the outcome measures of 'aids and adaptations', and 'dependency', because they correlated so closely with financial status, and employability.

11.4 DESCRIPTION OF COHORT

The intention of the series was to gather a cohort of patients who had survived severe brain damage. The patients were admitted consecutively over an 18-month period. Brain damage was originally defined as an injury which caused unconsciousness for more than an hour, or an interval of PTA lasting more than 24 hours. More than 12 years has now elapsed since the start of the study, and it is now standard to define severe head injury as one which has caused more than 6 hours unconsciousness, although 24 hours remains as the critical minimum for defining severe head injury in terms of PTA. It was decided for the final analysis to apply the more modern definitions. It also became apparent that some of the original patients had sustained brain damage but not from head injury, and that they should also be excluded from the figures (Table 11.4). Unfortunately, it proved impossible to see and fully examine all the cohort, so for some only the questionnaire was administered; in some cases this had to be done by post. Despite the difficulties only 7 out of the original 137 patients had no follow-up, all of whom had sustained mild injuries as far as could be judged by the duration of PTA and unconsciousness.

There were thus 94 remaining for subsequent study. They were examined fully where possible over a period of at least 24 hours. Where this was not possible a shorter examination was used, and in some case only a questionnaire or interview was possible (Table 11.5). The average time to follow-up was 4 years 9 months, the mode was 5 years (Figure 11.2). Tables 11.6 to 11.9 describe some of the characteristics of the patients in the cohort.

The duration of unconsciousness was found to be the most effective predictor of outcome; much better in this study than PTA. This was

Table 11.4 Reasons for exclusion from cohort

Reason	Number
Too mild	22
Not head injury	14
Traced, not seen	3
Not traced	3
No information	1
Total	43

Table 11.5 Methods used in follow-up

Method	Number
Full	64
Exam and questionnaire	14
Questionnaire only	11
Examination only	3
Interview only	2
Total	94

Table 11.6 Hand dominance

Dominant side	Number
Right handed	79
Left handed	13
Ambidextrous	2
Total	94

Table 11.7 Sex distribution

Sex	Number
Male	86
Female	8
Total	94

Table 11.8 Alcohol involvement

Alcohol	Number
Yes	22
No	47
Not recorded	25
Total	94

Table 11.9 Duration of unconsciousness

Unconscious time	Number
Severe	
<6 hours, but PTA >24 hours	3
>6 hours, <24 hours	10
>1 day, <2 days	4
Total severe	17
Very severe injury (>2 days unconscious)	
>2 days, <4 days	12
>4 days, <1 week	11
>1 week, <2 weeks	12
>2 weeks, <3 weeks	10
>3 weeks, <1 month	6
>1 month, <2 months	9
>2 months, <3 months	10
>3 months	4
Insufficient information	3
Total very severe	77
Total	**94**

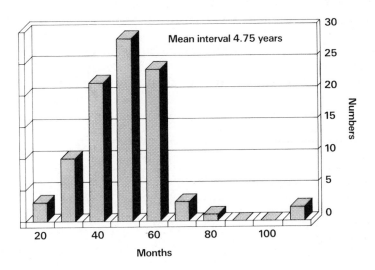

Figure 11.2 Head-injured patients: time from injury to review.

partly because the end point was more difficult to recognize, and partly because some of the patients were so severely injured that they could not be said to ever come out of PTA. It will be seen from Table 11.9 that all of the group had by definition sustained a severe head injury and that 77 of the 94 patients (79%) had sustained a very severe head injury as they had been seen to be unconscious for more than 48 hours (McLellan, 1987). It must be stressed, however, that while it may be possible to predict, for example, that 50% of patients who are unconscious for one week or less will get back to work it does not predict which individuals will do so.

As the results were analysed it also became apparent that if duration of unconsciousness was a successful measure of severity of lesion (although not infallible) then the most consistent outcome measure was employability. It related closely with financial status, independence and where and how the patient eventually lived, and the amount and extent of aids and adaptations needed.

11.5 OUTCOMES

Employability

It seemed at first that these data would be difficult to establish, but experience showed that with time and care accuracy was possible. Where there was ambiguity the Registrar General's classification of occupations (1970) was used. The list on p. 187 shows the categories of employment outcome, (a) to (g). In many of the tables and graphs which follow categories (a) and (b) are amalgamated, as are (e) and (f) (Table 11.10).

If there was doubt about the status of a job for Table 11.10 it was

Table 11.10 Categories of employability

Category	Number
Return to same or equivalent job	41
Unemployed	17
Return to a job of poorer status	11
Training (time elapsed)	4
Sheltered employment	3
Unemployable	18
Total	94

Table 11.11 Employability v unconscious time

Unconscious time	Same job	No job	Poorer job	Train/ sheltered	Unemployable
<1 h	2	1	0	0	0
>1 h, <1 day	12	0	0	0	0
>1 day, <3 days	9	3	1	0	0
>3 days, <1 week	10	2	2	1	0
>1 week, <2 weeks	6	6	2	1	0
>2 weeks, <1 month	1	5	4	2	4
>1 month, <2 months	0	0	2	1	6
>2 months, <3 months	1	0	0	2	6
>3 months	0	0	0	0	2
	41	17	11	7	18
Total					**94**

checked in HMSO Classification of Occupations. It will be seen that of this group of severely brain-damaged patients 41 out of 94 (43.6%) got back to their original or equivalent employment, and if those who were back at fulltime, though poorer-status employment are included then 52 out of 94 (55.3%) were capable of earning.

Table 11.11 shows the relationship between the duration of unconsciousness and category of employment at review in some detail and the information is also presented in greater detail in Figure 11.3.

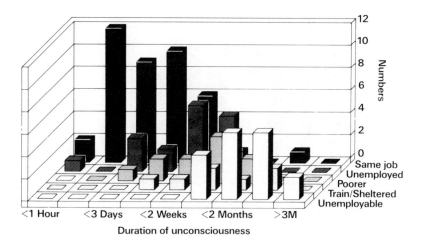

Figure 11.3 Employment outcome: duration of unconsciousness v category of employment attained.

It shows the gradual deterioration of employment prospects as the duration of unconsciousness increases. Surely a statement of the obvious, but it does set some attainable figures. It can be seen that no patient who was unconscious for less than 2 weeks was unemployable, and that one who had been unconscious for more than 2 months was back at his original job.

Finance

We expected some patients to be reluctant in revealing their earnings. For most part, however, the investigators felt that the answers given were honest, and are remarkably consistent. Details of the enquiries are included later, near the figures obtained. Figure 11.4 shows the annual income of families disclosed at the time of review but index linked to 1982. Unfortunately, there were gaps in the information, but this graph represents a fair sample. It shows the amount earned per earner (back row) and also the amount earned by each group in total and averaged (front row). It is not clear why those patients who were only slightly injured as judged by an unconscious time of less than 1 hour (although PTA was greater than 24 hours) should earn so little. But after this hiccup the deterioration of earning power is clearly seen.

Figure 11.5 takes this further. It shows the relationship between the duration of unconsciousness and the income of the patient (or his

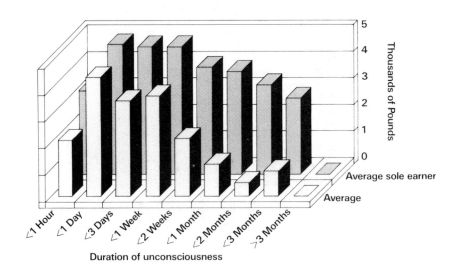

Figure 11.4 Financial outcome: duration of unconsciousness v annual income attained.

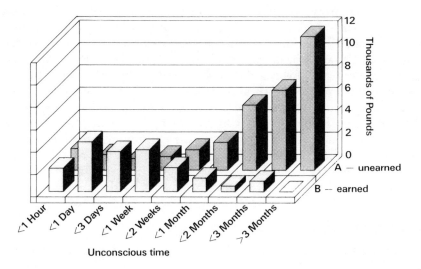

Figure 11.5 Families of head-injured patients: earned *v* unearned income (1982 rates).

family) and its source. It should be noted that the annual income recorded represents the income after tax coming into the household. Earned income is obvious but the unearned income could come from pension, compensation or DHSS allowance. Where a lump sum payment had been made it was estimated to produce an income of 10% of the capital for the patient. Where it was known that a patient was in residential care in a hospital or voluntary home a figure of £12 000 per annum has been added. More details about the five patients in this series who went into residential care are given later. All figures for income and accommodation have been calculated at 1982 values. They should be multiplied by 23.1% to bring them to 1987 equivalents.

It will be seen that until column 7 (unconscious for more than 1 month) is reached unearned income from whatever source is minimal. It becomes more important until the most severe category is reached when there is no earned income at all. It will be noted that in this series there are some earnings being made by patients up to column 8, i.e. those who had been unconscious for more than 2 months, but less than 3 months.

Impact of IQ

The relationship between the fall off in IQ was measured in the education department. Here the results of aptitude tests from recruit selection boards had been standardized with commercially available tests (Vivash, 1973). For this analysis a distinction was drawn between those who showed lower results than pre-injury and those with no significant change. This is a difference between the extremes. Of those who showed no decrease in ability on arrival at Chessington, 48.6% got back to their same or equivalent work whereas only 15% of those whose IQs had fallen did so. It also seemed, for those who were able to be followed-up, that this recovery was still taking place after some years had elapsed since the injury. This was confirmed by the reports from all the testing methods, and when the results were finally analysed, late changes were the rule rather than the exception.

Relationship of original job to re-employment

It has been suggested that there is a relationship between original type of employment and subsequent return to work. There were six categories of work differentiated by the survey; at the time of the reviews the present employment was examined, and then compared with that before the accident (Tables 11.12 and 11.13). It was found that neither of the professionals got back to their original work, nor any of those who had been in fulltime education, although two of the latter got poorer jobs. Those with clerical posts prior to the accident seemed to do better than average.

Epilepsy was found throughout all age groups and most durations of unconsciousness. It had a devastating effect on employability (Figure 11.6). This should be a statement of the obvious, but it cannot be all that obvious because there is no general policy for the use of

Table 11.12 Categories of employment after injury, and numbers

Category	Number
Manual unskilled	30
Manual semiskilled	24
Manual skilled	19
Clerical	9
Fulltime education	8
Professional	2
Other/not recorded	2
Total	**94**

Table 11.13 Return to work related to original employment

Category	Number	Same job	Same (%)	Poorer job	Numbers returned to work	Returned to work (%)
Manual unskilled	30	13	43.3	3	16.0	53.3
Manual semiskilled	24	9	37.5	4	13.0	54.2
Manual skilled	19	7	36.8	4	11.0	57.9
Clerical	9	6	66.7	1	7.0	77.8
Professional	2	0	0	1	1.0	50.0
Fulltime education	8	0	0	2	2.0	25.0
Not recorded	2					
	Total **94.0**		**Average** **46.1**		**Total** **50.0**	**Average** **53.0**

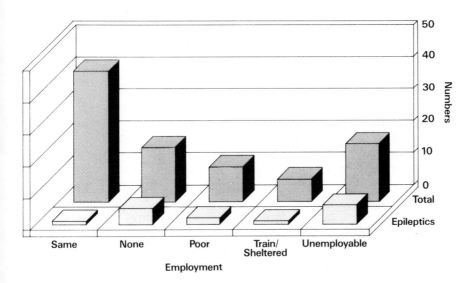

Figure 11.6 Impact of epilepsy: only 1 in 41 in the same job had epilepsy.

anti-convulsants after head injury; as Jennett (1985) points out there are no such universal guidelines published.

Social outcomes

Hobbies and pastimes

The questionnaire asked patients whether they had lost hobbies or social contact after the accident. The results were no surprise: there was a great fall off in activities undertaken, despite the difficulty in identifying hobbies for many. It was surprising how many listed pub and TV as their only hobbies or pastime! Driving and social contact were felt as major losses. Several patients expressed loss of confidence as a great problem too, many singling out loss of concentration and memory as contributing to their impoverishment. This correlated with observed outcomes.

Accommodation

Despite the severity of the injuries, only 5 patients were in residential care at the time of review. They were all patients who had been unconscious for 2 weeks or more. Half were in their family home, and this said much for the level of family commitment. Community rehabilitation services were patchy, and a lot of relatives expressed their desolation at their lot, but could not see how to get help.

11.6 CONCLUSIONS

Some conclusions can be drawn from the information from this study. First, that in order for any relevant assessments of patients in hospital to be made they need to be related to a practical outcome scale such as employability, financial status or dependency. Secondly, it is possible to give a closely defined social outcome, although it may appear to be invidious to compare a patient's achievements after head injury to those before. This is helpful, however, in planning rehabilitation since it is less likely to set targets which are unrealistically high (or low). Furthermore, a policy of finding out original social factors will help to avoid making a patient conform to the therapists' and doctors' mores and behaviour rather than the peer group from which the patient has come.

Other conclusions from this series which are quite surprising are that no patient who was unconscious for less than 3 days failed to get back to his or her original job. Indeed resumption of previous job was possible until unconsciousness lasted for more than 3 weeks. After this time no patients got back to their original or equivalent work. Only three patients earned money after this time span. No patient unconscious for 10 weeks or more earned any money at all. Of the five patients who 'cost' more than £12 000 per annum one had coeliac disease, but lived at home; all the others were in 'institutional care'. Only one patient unconscious for less than 3 days was a 'cost'. He was a swashbuckling character who had listed his hobbies before the head injury as 'rugby, football, swimming, pubs and women'. He saw no reason to change after the injury!

REFERENCES

Brooks, N. (1984) *Closed Head Injury. Psychological, Social and Family Consequences*, Oxford University Press.

Cairns, H. and Holbourn, H. (1943) Head Injuries in Motor Cyclists, *Brit. Med. J.*, **1**, 591–98.

Eames, P. and Wood, R. (1985a) Rehabilitation after Severe Head Injury: a special-unit approach to behaviour disorders. *Init. Rehabil. Med.*, **7**, 130–33.

Eames, P. and Wood, R. (1985b) Rehabilitation after Severe Brain Injury. A follow-up study of a behaviour modification approach. *J. Neurol. Neurosurg. Psychiat.*, **48**, 613–19.

Evans, C.D. *et al.* (1974) The Assessment of Disability Caused by Severe Head Injury. *Proc. R. Soc. Med.*, **67**, 486–88.

Evans, C.D. (1976) Rehabilitation of the Brain Damaged Survivor. *Injury*, **8**, 80.

Evans, C.D. (ed.) (1981) *Rehabilitation after Severe Head Injury*. Churchill Livingstone, Edinburgh.

Hooper, R.S. (1966) Head Injuries – Past, Present and Future, *Med. J. Austr.*, **2**, 45–53.

Jacobson, W.H.A. (1886) On Middle Meningeal Haemorrhage, *Guys Hospital Reports*, **43**, 147–308.

Jennett, B. and Teasdale, G. (1981) in *Management of Head Injuries*, F.A. Davies, Philadelphia.

Jennett, B. (1985) Epilepsy (2) — After Head Injury and Craniotomy in *Medical Aspects of Fitness to Drive* (A. Raffle, ed.), Medical Commission on Accident Prevention, London.

Knight, P.N. (1972) Rehabilitation of Head Injury. *Nursing Mirror*, March, 14–18.

Lewis, N.R. (1966) Rehabilitation after Head Injury. *Proc. Roy. Soc. Med.*, **59**, 623–35.

London, P.S. (1967) Some Observations in the Course of Events after Severe Head Injury. *Ann. R. Coll. Surg. Eng.*, **41**, 460.

London, P.S. (Chairman) (1988) *Report: A Rehabilitation Service for the West Midlands*, West Midland Regional Health Authority, Birmingham.

McLellan, D.L. (Chairman) (1988) *The Management of Traumatic Brain Injury*. Report of a Working Party of the Medical Disability Society.

Oppenheimer, D.R. (1968) *J. Neurol. Neurosurg. and Psych.*, **31**, 229–306.

Plum, F. and Posner, B. (1972) *Diagnosis of Stupor and Coma*, 2nd edn, F.A. Davis, Philadelphia.

Registrar General's Classification of Occupations (1970) HMSO, London.

Russell, W.R. (1964) Some Reactions of the Nervous System to Trauma, *Brit. Med. J.*, **2**, 403.

Stichbury, J.C. (1975) Assessment of Disability following Severe Head Injury. *Physiotherapy*, **61**, 268.

Stichbury, J.C., Davenport, M. and Middleton, F.R.I. (1980) Head-Injured Patients, a Combined Therapeutic Approach. *Physiotherapy*, **66**, 288–92.

Strich, S.J. (1956) *J. Neurol. Neurosurg. and Psychiat.*, **19**, 163–85.

Strich, S.J. (1961) *Lancet*, **ii**, 443–48.

Vivash, E.P. (1973) Assessment and Re-education at the Joint Services Medical Rehabilitation Unit, Chessington. *Services Education*, **1**, 9–11.

Wade, D.T. and Langton Hewer, R. (1987) Epidemiology of some Neurological Diseases (with special reference to workload on the NHS), *Int. Rehabil. Med.*, **8**, 129–37.

12 An information system to assess the effectiveness of brain injury rehabilitation

William J. Haffey and Mark V. Johnston

The past decade has witnessed a rapid proliferation of head injury rehabilitation programs in the United States. Rehabilitation services are now being provided to head injury survivors who previously were considered ineligible for traditional inpatient rehabilitation programmes. Such patient groups include persons in coma, persons with severe conduct disorders, and persons whose rate of change in functional skills was too limited to satisfy **utilization review criteria** for continued service provision in inpatient rehabilitation programmes. Expansion has been even more dramatic in the later stages of rehabilitation with the advent of service models designed to promote residential, occupational, and social readaptation.

The New Medico Head Injury System (NMHIS) has attempted to evaluate the effectiveness of a range of rehabilitation services. As a specialized system for brain injury rehabilitation it is a prime example of the expansion of head injury rehabilitation services in the US. In the 4-year period from September 1982 to September 1986, the NMHIS evolved from a single inpatient rehabilitation unit serving 15 patients to a system of 22 facilities serving 564 patients. These facilities provide a range of programmes including coma management, acute rehabilitation, non-hospital residential, transitional and community re-entry training, prevocational and vocational rehabilitation, outpatient rehabilitation, extended rehabilitation, long-term residential care, and respite services.

Brain injury rehabilitation is such a new field that there is a pressing need for research to validate and improve the effectiveness of its interventions. The Glasgow studies (Jennett and Bond, 1975; Jennett *et al.*, 1981; McKinlay *et al.*, 1981; Livingston *et al.*, 1985; Brooks *et al.*, 1986; 1987) are of long-term outcomes for brain-injured patients who have not received formal rehabilitation. There is now a body of research on prognosis after brain injury (Najenson *et al.*, 1975; Jennett *et al.*, 1976; Gilchrist and Wilkinson, 1979; Jennett *et al.*, 1979; Braakman *et al.*, 1980; Gianotta *et al.*, 1987) although prediction of outcomes in individual cases remains problematic. Studies examining the effectiveness of rehabilitative interventions with brain injury survivors are just beginning to appear (Prigatano *et al.*, 1984; Eames and Wood, 1985; Ben-Yishay *et al.*, 1985; Scherzer, 1986; Ben-Yishay *et al.*, 1987; Fryer and Haffey, 1987).

The New Medico Office of Research was established in February, 1985. Its chief mandate was to develop and implement a study of the outcomes of brain injury after rehabilitation. The outcome study evolved into an investigation of the effectiveness and efficiency of New Medico's brain injury rehabilitation programmes. The first phase of the outcome study was the development of a comprehensive set of tools to assess the effectiveness of rehabilitation for brain-injured persons.

Taken together these tools are known as the **Rehabilitation Effectiveness Information System** (REIS). The central and largest element of the REIS is the **Comprehensive Assessment Inventory for Rehabilitation** (CAIR). The CAIR is employed by clinicians to describe clients' health and physical, neurobehavioural, and psychological functioning in the treatment setting. A major feature of the CAIR is its ability to link patient disabilities or functional status to the impairments underlying them. The CAIR is closely linked to the **Pre-injury History and Social Support Questionnaire**, which contains information on client functioning before the injury or disease and on current social support, and to the **case management information system**, which describes specific treatment goals and the human resources which were expended towards each of these primary goals. The **Rehabilitation Outcome Questionnaire** collects data on the ultimate outcome of rehabilitation. Its major feature is the attempt to gather information not only on disability but also on handicap – the disadvantage or subjective burden that clients and family experience in the post-discharge environment. The **financial management information system** is linked to these data bases to permit study of cost-effectiveness.

This chapter describes the set of instruments which comprise the REIS, the concepts which underlie it, and its intended uses and its implementation.

12.1 CONCEPTUAL FRAMEWORK

The development of the REIS began by reviewing methods currently employed to assess the effectiveness of rehabilitation after head injury. The result was a dissatisfaction with most measures for a variety of reasons. Some of the reasons were logistical. For example, it was determined that it was not economically feasible to have patients and families return to clinical centres for longitudinal follow-up due to the geographical spread of the population served. Other reasons were conceptual. Clinical experience led us to agree with Hart and Hayden's (1986) conclusion that 'standard neuropsychological tests may have limited ecological validity when they are used as outcome measures for rehabilitation after closed head injury' (p. 205), a conclusion also reached by Wood (1987). To develop a satisfactory approach, we returned to the conceptual foundations of rehabilitation.

The current conception of rehabilitation for persons with an acquired injury or disorder is that rehabilitation is a process designed to yield 'readaptation to community living' (Frey, 1984; p. 11). In his historical overview of the functional assessment movement, Frey noted that the curative medicine model proved inadequate as a conceptual foundation for rehabilitation. Rehabilitative interventions are designed primarily to reduce the impact or consequences of disease or impairments rather than to decrease the disease or impairment *per se*.

Realization of this fundamental difference between curative medicine and rehabilitation led to the development of alternative conceptual models, of which Nagi's (1969) and Wood's (1975) are prime examples. Wood's model was incorporated into *International Classification of Impairments, Disabilities, and Handicaps* (WHO, 1980). In this taxonomy, **impairment** exists at an organ or organ system level and represents anatomical, physiological, or psychological loss, abnormality, or injury. **Disability** encompasses a loss or limitation of a person's ability to perform an activity or task. **Handicap** is concerned with the disadvantage or social consequence which the individual experiences due to these impairments and disabilities and is specified in terms of limitation on fulfilment of roles normally associated with the individual's age, sex, and sociocultural group.

The Wood–WHO conceptualization is the guiding framework for development of the REIS. As it stands, the REIS may be described as attempt to realize Wood–WHO concepts and adapt them for brain injury rehabilitation. Unlike previous instruments, the REIS attempts to systematically assess clients at all three levels – impairment, disability, and handicap.

Throughout the development of the REIS, certain beliefs or

principles regarding rehabilitation effectiveness and its measurement guided our decisions:

1. The behaviours sampled should be comprehensive enough to indicate the impact of the brain injury on the individual's and family's life experiences (Levin, 1985, p. 296);
2. The aim of rehabilitation is reduction in problems at the level of life activities and values – disability and handicap. Reduction in impairment is an important means to this end, but it is not an end in itself or the only way by which disability or handicap can be reduced;
3. Reduction in handicap is the ultimate outcome to patients and family, not reduction in disability alone;
4. Impairments must be measured to understand treatment efficacy;
5. Performance in the discharge environment is a more relevant indicator of outcome than performance in the treatment setting;
6. Observed performance rather than capacity or ability is the criterion of interest.

The goal: impact on life experience

The first three principles are intertwined. Rehabilitation aims at affecting the life experience and activities of the disabled person and his or her family or significant others. It is not possible to assess the effectiveness of rehabilitation without measures that tap each of the major domains which rehabilitation aims to affect.

Rehabilitation outcomes cannot be assessed at the level of impairments. Impairments are so numerous that they cannot be combined to gain any overall impression of the effectiveness of non-curative interventions. Reduction of disability and handicap is the *sine qua non* of rehabilitation.

Beyond disability: Handicap

Although disability reduction is associated with handicap reduction, it is not the only way by which handicap can be reduced. Handicap (the disadvantage experienced as a consequence of impairments and disabilities) can for instance be reduced by altering environmental demands without change in the person's performance level. Psychological interventions can reduce the distress experienced by clients and families without significant change in the performance levels of the patient. Provision of a functional skill which does not reduce the burden or distress which clients experience or which proves impractical is pointless.

Handicap, as opposed to disability, is particularly salient with brain-injured populations. Problems performing activities of daily living (ADL) or other specific tasks are frequently not the main sources of distress to such patients and family in the long run. Rather, problems with behavioural control, cognition, emotion, and personality change are most frequently reported as the main sources of stress by patients and relatives (Weddell et al., 1980; Levin et al., 1982; Brooks, 1984; Lezak, 1987; Livingston, 1987). These problems do not fit easily into traditional disability paradigms, which are oriented towards physical activities. To brain injury survivors and those close to them, handicap reduction is the desired rehabilitation outcome. To estimate the effectiveness of rehabilitation, one must measure handicap.

Measuring handicap

Many well-developed disability measures (i.e. functional assessment measures) can be found in rehabilitation. The same cannot be said of handicap measures (Granger and Gresham, 1984; Halpern and Fuhrer, 1984). One approach which at least reflects handicap is found in conventional indicators such as employment status, income, family role status, and living arrangement. Such status indicators summarize the interaction of disability and environment after discharge and are clearly essential to characterize the ultimate outcomes of rehabilitation. Status indicators are included in the REIS.

In the Wood–WHO framework, handicap encompasses six dimensions of human experience which are labeled **survival roles**. These are: orientation, physical independence, mobility, occupation, social integration, and economic self-sufficiency. The REIS assesses these as global disabilities in the Rehabilitation Outcome Questionnaire. Disabilities which would not be applicable to a person under normal circumstances are excluded (e.g. lack of employment is not a handicap for those who are retired or are independently wealthy).

Such general indicators appear, however, to be fairly indirect or insensitive as measures of handicap. What is most distinctive about handicap, as opposed to disability, is that handicap has to do with *valuation* of the *consequences* of disability. With general handicap indicators, the valuation is inferred by the researcher on the basis of putative social norms. While this is undoubtedly a useful and even essential procedure, in a culture as heterogeneous as that in the US, serious questions can be raised about specifying values on the basis of 'norms'. Our experience with brain-injured patients and their families after discharge from rehabilitation led us to conclude that status indicators alone are insensitive to important differences in the experiences and values of individuals served.

We decided that handicap might be best assessed by asking the brain injury survivor, and those close to him or her, directly about the burden or distress they experience related to different domains of function (McKinlay et al., 1981). These questions are put to clients and families after discharge in the Rehabilitation Outcome Questionnaire. Clinical experience indicates that long-term and episodic stress appear to be primary contributors to breakdown of the family support system and to subsequent institutionalization.

This approach taps directly into the matter of valuation of the consequence of disability and provides information not available from other attempts to deal with handicap. Rehabilitation professionals already know a great deal about the clients' disabilities and discharge status, but they typically are less certain about which of the skills they impart will be most valued by clients in the long run. Our approach to handicap will enable us to provide treatment professionals with such information.

Impairments

A powerful factor which guided the development of data collection instruments was the desire to link disabilities to impairments. The motivation behind this linkage was the intent to compare the effectiveness and efficiency of alternative treatment strategies. For example, the relative effectiveness and efficiency of a traditional functional training regime by physical therapy can be properly compared with a Neurodevelopmental Programming approach only if the underlying reasons for the disability are roughly equivalent. To compare a group for whom muscle weakness is the principal impairment to one for whom impaired kinesthetic feedback is the principal barrier to effective ambulation would be pointless in this context.

Impairments must be measured not because rehabilitation aims at impairment reduction as an end in itself but because it is not possible to understand why a clinical intervention is effective in one case but ineffective in another unless impairments are assessed.

Follow-up

Our fifth principle – that performance in the discharge environment is a more relevant indicator of outcome than performance in the treatment setting – is shared by many others in rehabilitation (e.g. Brown et al., 1982; Hart and Hayden, 1986; Wood, 1987). The aim of rehabilitation is not merely to improve patient functioning in the treatment setting but to improve patient functioning in the community after discharge. From the standpoint of benefits to patient and society, a rehabilitation programme that improves patient functioning in the treatment setting but not after discharge is indistinguishable from a care or maintenance programme. The follow-up measure is the chief vehicle for assessing performance and handicap in the discharge environment.

Observed performance

Underlying all measurement in the REIS is the belief that observed performance, rather than capacity or ability, is the criterion of greatest interest (see Brown *et al.*, 1982; Wood, 1987). There are two reasons for this.

First, the measurement of rehabilitation outcomes must be based on observed behaviour to ensure reliability and objectivity. Inferred or judged ability or benefit are not credible bases for scientific research. Observed behaviour in the treatment setting is a test of performance which is appropriate and practical for rehabilitation. However, such a test may show maximal rather than typical performance. It may also be setting-specific. This is why assessment of performance in the discharge setting is essential.

Second, the capactiy to perform a task, in the absence of actual performance, contributes minimally to altering experienced disadvantage or handicap. Handicap is related to performance in everyday life situations.

We will now illustrate how we have attempted to put these principles into operation.

12.2 THE COMPREHENSIVE ASSESSMENT INVENTORY FOR REHABILITATION

The Comprehensive Assessment Inventory for Rehabilitation (CAIR) describes patient disabilities and the impairments which give rise to these disabilities. Functional assessment measures currently employed in rehabilitation are, with few exceptions, disability measures. Existing impairment measures were not constructed with the aim of linking them with disability or handicap. The CAIR was constructed to identify the relationship between a given disability and the factors (impairments and other disabilities) which contribute to it.

A unique feature of the CAIR is the scaling of impairments not according to their physiological intensity (severity *per se*) but according to the degree to which they typically interfere with activities in the person's life. This method was chosen primarily because it makes the rating maximally relevant to disability and handicap reduction and permits an analysis of the relative significance of the impairment to rehabilitative outcomes.

Selection of the CAIR content domains was guided by our belief that the behaviours sampled should be comprehensive enough to indicate the impact of the brain injury on the life of the individual and his or her family (Levin, 1985, p. 296). Since our brain injury population ranges from patients in coma to persons preparing for community readaptation, the CAIR had to have items reflecting the issues confronted by individuals at all points in the recovery continuum.

Domains of relevance were selected by examining the research literature on head injury outcomes (e.g. Najenson *et al.*, 1978; Bowers and Marshall, 1980; Najenson *et al.*, 1975; Weddell *et al.*, 1980; Brooks, 1984; Thomsen, 1984; Levin, 1985; and Oddy *et al.*, 1985). Items were developed primarily by Haffey to measure patient function in the relevant domains. These were submitted to clinicians with a minimum of 5 years experience in head trauma rehabilitation for review. Data forms and content were field tested by having physicians, licensed nurses, allied health professionals, nursing aides, and residential staff rate 10 patients in coma intervention programmes, 10 patients in acute rehabilitation programmes, and 9 patients in residential community re-entry programmes. Each respondent was debriefed after completing the inventory to elicit reactions to the relevance of the content domains and items.

The content domains which were eventually selected (Table 12.1) will now be discussed in turn. (The inventory reflects labels employed in the WHO'S *International Classification.*)

Physical health impairments

Physical health is often cited as one of the most basic qualities of life in surveys of the general population (Flanagan, 1982) and in conceptual formulations of quality of life for a disabled individual (Trieschmann, 1974; Kottke, 1982). Prevention of medical complications is especially salient for comatose persons. The CAIR includes nine areas of 'organismic' health which are often problematic for severely head-injured persons. These areas are respiration, infections, fevers of an undetermined source, skin breakdowns, blood pressure irregularities/abnormalities, seizures, hydrocephalus, sustaining adequate levels of nutrition and hydration, and heterotopic bone

Table 12.1 Content domains of the comprehensive
assessment inventory for rehabilitation

Physical health impairments
Impairments in global environmental responsivity
Self-care and mobility disabilities
Residential-community ADL disabilities
Musculoskeletal and body movement impairments
Impairment of attention
Ocular, aural, and sensory impairments
Impairment of perception
Impairment of memory
Communicative disabilities
Impairments of language and speech functions
Impairments of thinking
Awareness of disabilities
Impairments of emotive functions
Impairment of behaviour pattern

Table 12.2 Restriction on activities scale

---

0 Typically no restriction on activity levels
1 Typically only places restriction on strenuous
  exercises
2 Typically places limits on activity level, but does
  not inhibit participation in usual therapy sessions
3 Typically limits participation in usual therapy
  sessions
4 Typically requires close monitoring but does not
  restrict person to bed or chair
5 Requires restriction to bed or chair

---

formations. An open-ended category for all other medical/physical
health complications concludes the content area in this section.

For each content area, the intensity of problems over the last 2
weeks is rated on a multipoint scale and instances of the problem are
specified. In a few areas, the severity of the physical problem *per se* is
rated (e.g. skin breakdown). In most cases, intensity is scaled by the
impact of the problem on life activities. For example, after reporting
the nature of problems with maintaining normal blood pressure, a
selection is made from the six-point 'restriction on activities' scale in
Table 12.2.

Global environmental responsivity
General responsiveness to the environment is an issue unique to brain injury patients. The next section of the CAIR consists of the Glasgow Coma Scale (Jennett and Bond, 1975) and the Rancho Los Amigos Scale of Cognitive Functioning (Hagen, Malkmus, and Durham, 1974). If the person is rated at Rancho levels, I, II, or III, the respondent has completed the items which pertain to this patient. Individuals at these levels are so severely impaired that they are presumed to be totally disabled in the remaining domains contained in the CAIR.

Self-care and mobility disabilities

So much work has been done refining measures of functional independence in self-care and mobility ADLs in acute rehabilitation settings (e.g. Granger and Gresham, 1984) that invention of totally new scales was unnecessary. Scale content and physical assistance levels were derived from the **Functional Independence Measure** (FIM) developed by the Task Force for Development of a Uniform Data System (UDS) for Medical Rehabilitation (Granger *et al.*, 1986). Disability in self-care ADLs is rated with five items. Toileting is rated with three items, and mobility, with 13. The toileting section also contains items dealing with frequency of bowel and bladder incontinence, equipment and special procedures and impairments involved with meeting elimination needs.

Traditional functional measures scale disability by the level or amount of assistance required to complete a given task. The scales used in this assessment employ this principle but depart from traditional measures by separating physical assistance from cognitive assistance, that is, supervision and verbal assistance. This was done because cognitive problems requiring supervision and cueing are pre-eminent problems with brain-injured persons. The assumption of traditional US functional status scales – that supervision is less burdensome than physical assistance – is questionable with a brain-injured population.

The physical assistance and the cognitive assistance scales we employ are depicted in Tables 12.3 and 12.4. With the exception of supervision/cognitive assistance, scale levels differ from those in the National Data System only in numeric abbreviation; the content of levels is the same. As a consequence, findings from these scales can be compared to findings from centres which employ the National Data System using a computer score conversion process.

Table 12.3 Physical assistance scale

Rate the typical level of physical assistance given using the numeric codes below. When component behaviours require varying levels of assistance, rate the *maximal* degree of assistance *typically* needed to complete the total activity.

0.0 *Complete independence of physical help.* Activity typically performed within reasonable time without physical assistance from others and without assistive devices.

1.0 *Limited/modified independence.* Task completed without *any* physical assistance from others. Device/equipment used independent of physical assistance. Extra time may be required. Any safety (risk) considerations do not require supervision by others.

Helper/dependent levels:

2.0 *Set-up only.* Caregiver helps at one point, typically by setting up adaptive equipment or materials. S/he then leaves and the task is completed without further *physical* assistance.

2.3 *Standby*/contact guard. Close standby. No more help than touching.

2.5 *Minimal physical assistance.* Caregiver does no more than 25% of physical activity (10-25%).

2.7 *Minimal-moderate assistance.* Caregiver does somewhat less than half of physical activity (25%-40%).

3.0 *Moderate physical assistance.* Caregiver does about 50% of physical activity necessary to perform the task (40%-60%).

3.5 *Moderate-maximal assistance.* Caregiver does somewhat more than half of physical activity (60%-75%).

4.0 *Maximal assistance of one person.* Caregiver does 75% or more of the activity. Patient does usefully perform part of physical activity.

4.5 *Maximal physical assistance of two* or more persons. Patient does small part of physical activity.

5.0 *Totally physically unable.* The activity has to be physically performed by others, with no contribution from the injured person.

If person not tested, use abbreviations below to express your best judgement. Use these rather than leaving items blank.

I Not tested, most likely *independent*/modified independence (0.0-1.0)
S Not tested, most likely *slight/some dependence* (2.0-2.5)
M Not tested, most likely *moderately dependent* (2.7-3.5)
UM Not tested, most likely *unable/maximum dependence* (4.0-5.0)

Residential-community ADL disabilities

The emergence of rehabilitative programmes focusing on residential and community reintegration necessitated expansion of the content area typically contained in hospital functional assessment measures. Eight domains of household and community survival skills were defined: clothing management, shopping, meal preparation, kitchen

Table 12.4 Cognitive assistance scale

Rate typical level of verbal and cueing assistance (verbal encouragement, verbal or non-verbal cueing) and supervision required to complete activities. Cognitive assistance is informational assistance or encouragement. It is usually non-physical, but physical means (e.g. a touching gesture) or physical objects (e.g. cue cards) may be used to communicate information. Cognitive assistance may be given to help a person compensate for physical problems (e.g. instruction on how to walk with a walker) or for cognitive/motivational problems.

0.0 CI *Complete independence.* Tasks are completed safely and in reasonable time without cueing/encouragement/supervision from others or special devices to provide informational/cognitive assistance.

1.0 MI *Modified independence.* Completes task without assistance from others in a specially structured setting or with use of compensatory devices/equipment for informational/cognitive assistance. Extra time or effort may be required; supervision is not required for safe task completion.

2.0 SU *Set-up/cueing to initiate.* Verbal cues/encouragements are used at one point, typically to get person to begin the task. Caregiver can then leave and task is completed without further assistance. Caregiver may check on person once or twice thereafter (e.g. near expected conclusion).

2.5 Min *Minimal cognitive assistance: occasional cueing/verbal assistance or constant supervision.* Cueing/encouragement needed periodically throughout the task, but substantial effort is not required of the caregiver. Caregiver typically can leave during task perfomance for a short while.

2.7 MnM *Minimal–moderate cognitive assistance.* Same as above, but someone must typically be present throughout the task to provide supervision or cognitive assistance for safety/technique/encouragement.

3.0 Mod *Moderate assistance: frequent cueing/encouragement or great effort is intermittently required of the caregiver* (e.g. to overcome resistance). Caregiver must be present throughout the task. Patient contributes actively rather than simply responding to directions/cues/prompts. Alternatively, reinforcement is provided after completion of several components of the activity.

4.0 Max *Maximum cognitive assistance: constant cueing/encouragement needed throughout task.* The caregiver guides the patient to task completion using step-by-step directives or continuous verbal support. Patient completes task by following these directives/by responding to support. Alternatively, reinforcement is provided after completion of every component of the functional activity.

4.5 AU *Almost totally unable/unwilling.* Despite maximal cueing/verbal support, patient completes only part of task. The rest of the task must be physically completed by others.

5.0 TU *Totally unable/willing.* Virtually no part of the task can be completed even if continuous/maximal non-physical assistance were given. Task has to be done by others. No cues may be given because they would be useless or impractical.

NA *Not applicable.* Cognitive ability/assistance is irrelevant due to the physical barrier (e.g. quadriplegia as a barrier to walking). Use this rating only for cases where person is 5.0 in physical assistance.

If person not tested, uses abbreviations below to express your best judgement. Use these rather than leaving an item blank.

I Not tested, most likely *independent*/modified independence (0.0–1.5)
S Not tested, most likely *slight/some* dependence (2.0–2.5)
M Not tested, most likely *moderately* dependent (2.7–3.0)
UM Not tested, most likely *unable/maximum* dependence (4.0–5.0)

upkeep, household upkeep, money and time management, and consumer protection. Each of these is rated according to the degrees of physical assistance and supervision/verbal assistance required for completion of the activity using the scales in Tables 12.3 and 12.4.

Musculoskeletal and body movement impairments

The next section of the CAIR is designed to assess the impairments which give rise to the individual's need for physical assistance to perform everyday living activities. The rater is first asked to assess the global impact of musculoskeletal and body-movement impairments on performance of everyday life activities using the scale listed in Table 12.5. The rater then reports the extent to which 16 specific impairments (e.g. spasticity, paresis, limited range of motion) typically interfere with task performance in training situations. A six-point scale is used to rate the severity of the impairments which impede limb and truncal functioning.

We found it convenient to place brain-based motoric impairments, which manifest themselves in the musculoskeletal and body movement domain, in this section. Examples of such items include: problems in directing, controlling, or coordinating gross motor movements and rate of movement too fast for effective functioning.

Table 12.5 Musculoskeletal impairment impact scale

0 Impairment not present or, if present, has no impact on completing tasks or on the quality of task performance.

1 Impairment does not prevent performance, but assisting or adaptive devices may be needed or the quality of task performance is typically mildly to moderately deficient.

2 Impairment may occasionally prevent task performance even when assistive or adaptive devices are used and quality of task performance is typically mildly to moderately deficient.

3 Impairment may occasionally prevent task performance and quality of task performance is severely deficient.

4 Impairment typically prevents task performance, but in restricted circumstances a few tasks can typically be performed even though quality of performance is severely deficient.

5 Impairment virtually always prevents task performance.

Cognitive and communicative functioning

The next sections in the CAIR deal with cognitive and communicative functioning as follows: attention and concentration, elementary sensory processing, perception, learning and memory, verbal/non-oral expressive communication, reading comprehension, comprehension of spoken and written communications, decision making and problem solving, and adjusting for limitations. Two aspects of each disability/impairment are examined – its nature and its impact on performance. Each section begins with a question which directs the respondent to rate the global impact of the disability/impairment on life activities. If a negative impact is indicated, the nature and extent of any impairments involved are specified.

The phrase 'disability/impairment' is used here because in the domain of cognitive function the distinction between impairments and disabilities bcomes exceedingly fine or controversial. Is cognition an organ function, subservient to gratification of instrumental needs, or is it an end in itself? Advocates of both positions can be found. Given the current climate of opinion in brain injury rehabilitation, there is no choice but to measure communication and cognition both in themselves and as instruments to other life functions.

The four sections dealing with communication each begin with a global impact item which is structured in the same way as the impact scale presented in Table 12.5. The rater then reports the frequency of communicative disability across a range of situations in which the person has to perform to meet the demands of daily life. These ratings are designed to reflect the variability in communicative effectiveness as a function of the nature of the situational demand and other environmental factors. Had the rating been applied to a single communicative situation, it would present severe problems since crucial situational variables would not be held constant. In the expressive communication section, examples of these situations include:

1. expressing basic needs/desires
2. expressing oneself in social conversation
3. expressing oneself to personnel in a store or bank
4. expressing oneself to teachers or supervisors

These situations make it possible to follow clients longitudinally and assess communicative problems ranging from those which are typical immediately post-coma to those encountered by those preparing for return to community living and employment.

The respondent would then describe the relative contribution of

Table 12.6 Communication barriers scale

---

0 No barrier to communicative effectiveness
1 Minor barrier to communicative effectiveness (reduced efficiency only)
2 Moderate barrier to communicative effectiveness (ineffective up to 25% of the time)
3 Major barrier to communicative effectiveness (ineffective 25-75% of the time)
4 Nearly total barrier to communicative effectiveness (ineffective more than 75% of the time)
C Severe confusion precludes evaluation (do not use for cognitive impairments item)

---

various impairments to the person's communicative disability. In the expressive communication section, eight specific classes of impairment are rated using the scale contained in Table 12.6. Examples of these impairment classes are: apraxia; dysprosody; cognitive impairments; pragmatic deficits.

Not every section in the cognitive functioning portion of the CAIR is as detailed as the expressive communication section. In other sections, the global question examines the impact of attention or learning and memory on the person's overall performance and is followed by less detailed specification of situations or related impairments.

Awareness of disability

Rehabilitation personnel are virtually uniform in their endorsement of the need for a rating of a brain-injured survivor's awareness of disability, but there is little agreement about how to define such awareness in practice. We have chosen to examine the extent to which the individual actually makes adjustments in performance to satisfy situational task demands. The gradations of disability (Table 12.7) are based on how most persons in discharge environments would likely classify a person's performance, as contrasted to how rehabilitation professionals might grade the person's disability.

Impairments of emotive functions

Measurement of an individual's internal state (feelings, thoughts, beliefs, judgements etc.) has been the focus of research from the earliest days of clinical psychiatry and psychology. We decided that instead of inferring a person's internal state, we would examine specific behaviours which are associated with various psychiatric and psychological syndromes (e.g. depression, anxiety, phobia, mania,

Table 12.7 Awareness impact scale

0 No impact	The person modifies his/her task performance approach to compensate for residual impairments/disabilities to such an extent that s/he meets virtually all situational demands in ways that are consistent with non-disabled peers.
1 Mild impact	The person relies on methods that are different from non-disabled peers due to his/her need to compensate for residual impairments/disabilities. S/he employs such alternative methods/strategies successfully enough to meet virtually all situational demands, although reduced efficiency may be evident.
2 Moderate impact	Problems with recognizing the need to modify one's performance to compensate for residual impairments/disabilities prevent the person from meeting minimal performance standards in one important area of everyday life.
3 Severe impact	Problems with recognizing the need to modify one's performance to compensate for residual impairments/disabilities prevent acceptable performance in several important areas of everyday life.
4 Very severe impact	Problems with recognizing the need to modify one's performance to compensate for residual impairments/disabilities prevent acceptable performances in most important areas of everyday life.
5 Total impact	The person's lack of awareness of the need to modify one's performance to compensate for residual impairments/disabilities is so severe that virtually all areas of everyday life are impaired.

schizophrenia, paranoia, and so forth). For each of the 21 behavioural symptoms, data are gathered using a five-point frequency scale. This section is preceded by a global scale which examines the extent to which these symptomatic behaviours have typically interfered with everyday life activities. This approach has limitations, but we are most interested in the effect of rehabilitation on the individual's everyday life. Two brain-injured patients may have comparable levels of affective disorder as measured by the MMPI or Beck's Depression Index but one may be coping more successfully than the other.

Rehabilitation includes methods designed to reduce the person's affective disorder. The success of these interventions is assessed by the degree to which they affect activities demanded by everyday life. We recognize that a person's subjective experience can be enhanced without any consequential alteration in meeting the demands of everyday life. To assess this experience, a patient's self-report on these items is conducted when possible.

Impairment of behaviour pattern

Disruption of behavioural control is a major management problem of clinical staff and is often the greatest barrier to successful community readaptation of many severely injured survivors. Nine maladaptive verbal behaviours and 14 maladaptive physical actions are examined. Each category also has an open-ended 'other' category to capture idiosyncratic maladaptive behaviours which are not typical of brain-injured survivors. Each disordered behaviour is rated on a five-point scale of frequency. The impact of the *worst* single episode on those in the environment is then rated using the Social Behaviour Disruption Scale in Table 12.8. This method was chosen because staff and family members often characterize severity by the extent to which their lives and routines are disrupted by the behaviour. The worst instance is a key factor in determining level of subjective burden and may determine whether staff or family members will tolerate the head-injury survivor's presence in the setting. The simplicity of rating a single event rather than the mean or median should increase reliability.

We have also included an eliciting circumstances coding system (see Table 12.9) which allows the rater to indicate the nature of the antecedent conditions which have been typically associated with the

Table 12.8 Social behaviour disruption scale

Rate the *worst* single instance of this behaviour over the past 2 weeks.

0 None	The behaviour has not occurred.
1 Mildly disruptive	The behaviour is situationally inappropriate but does not overtly interfere with other persons' activities/routines.
2 Moderately disruptive	The behaviour interrupts normal ongoing environmental activities or routines, but resumption of these activities/routines is accomplished with little or no effort on the part of others. No risk of physical harm/danger to anyone or anything.
3 Severely disruptive	The behaviour is so disruptive that restoration of normal ongoing activities/routines is accomplished only when people in the setting spend a good deal of time/effort to manage the behaviour. No actual physical harm/injury to any person.
4 Very severely disruptive	The behaviour involves some harm/injury or poses unacceptable threat of physical harm/injury. Person has to be removed from the setting and/or chemical/physical restraints must be employed.
5 Totally disruptive	The behaviour is so extreme that discharge to a special secure facility was/is required.

Table 12.9 Eliciting circumstances codes

---

1 Person-specific
2 Task/behavioral demand-specific
3 Both multiple persons and multiple tasks – some specificity shown
4 Multiple persons and multiple tasks – little specificity shown
5 Generalized/indiscriminant
6 Drug/alcohol/medication effect
7 Menstrual period
8 Sleep disorder effect
9 Unclear/unknown

---

occurrence of each type of disordered behaviour. Information on eliciting circumstances is as important to understanding socially-maladaptive behaviour as impairment data are to understanding physical disability.

Trieschmann (1974) observed that a critical survival skill is the disabled individual's ability to maintain harmony with those responsible for providing care and assistance. In addition, prosocial behaviour is extremely important because people are much more forgiving of socially unacceptable behaviour when a person demonstrates prosocial behaviour at other times. Client status in general cooperation and the typical incidence of prosocial behaviour are both rated using a seven-point scale.

Implementation of the CAIR

The CAIR is based on observations and formal assessments conducted during the first 2 weeks after admission to and the last 2 weeks before discharge from each rehabilitation programme. For most rehabilitation candidates, it can also serve to describe change between periodic team conferences. All relevant items of the CAIR are completed at admission and discharge. Between these two points in time, the team records only changes in client functioning.

The CAIR is designed to be an integral part of routine clinical evaluation and record keeping. It provides a common framework and a common vocabulary for describing patient status, thus facilitating communication within and across teams within a facility, as well as across facilities. At the same time, no method of evaluating an individual's functioning is proscribed, and it is recognized that clinicians will need to use additional measurement tools for certain problems. Integration of the CAIR into the clinical record-keeping system overcomes problems that duplicate record-keeping systems typically engender, such as high rates of missing data and low reliability. Administrative support for duplicate record-keeping systems is typically lukewarm, at best, due to the additional expense.

The entire rehabilitation team is responsible for data collection. The CAIR has been designed to be segmented, with specific individuals having primary accountability for various items. Designation of these accountabilities is determined by the treatment personnel and their supervisors. Two reasons dictated this choice. First, not every clinical programme is organized in the same manner. Second, extensive reliability studies of earlier versions of the inventory revealed that no one class of reporters (disciplines) was unequivocally superior to other classes of reporters in most of the domains of patient functioning contained in the CAIR.

12.3 OTHER ELEMENTS OF REIS

The Case Management Information System

The Case Management Information System (CMIS) describes specific treatment goals and the human resources (treatment units) which were expended towards each of these goals. Goals are couched in terms of achievement of an observable improvement in patient functioning as measured by items in the CAIR. Projected discharge destination, projected and actual length of stay, anticipated payment sources, and other matters are also specified in the CMIS.

The source of data on projected goals is the **Client Service Plan**, a document communicated to payment sources and, when appropriate, with referral sources, clients, and families. In the US health care system, payment for services rendered is tied to documentation of patient progress. Consequently the projected goals in the case management system are very real, in the sense that real consequences are attached to success or failure to attain the goals.

Information on specific therapeutic goals for individuals makes possible analysis of the effectiveness of specific therapeutic modalities and judgement of the success or failure of a therapeutic intervention for an individual.

Pre-injury history and social support questionnaire

This questionnaire gathers information on patient and family functioning prior to the current trauma or disease and on the current social support available to clients. It is ordinarily administered to client and family by the social worker as a structured interview in the initial psychosocial intake, but it can be given by phone or mailed, if the family cannot be physically present.

There is every reason to believe that pre-injury history factors are significant predictors of outcome. The questionnaire emphasizes conditions that may constrain rehabilitation outcomes (e.g. history of learning disability, addictive drug use). More generally, we are interested in gaining an overview of the activity patterns of the client before the injury; previous employment history, education, and so on are recorded.

Available social support is a crucial predictor of discharge destination and support costs among severely disabled stroke victims (Johnston, 1983, for example). Similarly many brain-injured survivors will require continued care for years after the injury. Key indicators of the strength of the brain-injury survivor's social support system are included.

Deviation from pre-injury performance levels and statuses is an outstanding criterion by which head-injury survivors and family members judge the quality of their recovery and benefit from rehabilitation. It is important to assessment of handicap. The questionnaire attempts to provide a macro-view of the previous life experience of the patients and family so that the success of rehabilitation may be assessed as deviations from such experience.

Field Evaluator's Report

The *Field Evaluator's Report* is completed on candidates before admission. It documents factors relating to the nature and severity of the injury, to the patient's course in neurotrauma treatment centres, and other factors. The primary data source for the Field Evaluator's Report is the patient's medical record, supplemented by information obtained verbally from neurotrauma personnel and the family. The Field Evaluator's Report is used to screen candidates for safety and appropriateness of admission to rehabilitation and is a primary source of data for studies of the kind of facility and treatments which have the best potential for achieving desired outcomes.

Financial Management Information System

The *Financial Management Information System* (FMIS) documents charges, payment sources, actual revenue, and other factors associated with rehabilitation services. Linkage of other data bases with the FMIS is essential for research comparing the cost-effectiveness of alternative rehabilitative programmes and treatments. These data are essential in the US health-care system in which the continued survival of a treatment facility is linked to its economic health.

Rehabilitation outcome questionnaire

Assessment of the effectiveness of rehabilitation programmes must include an investigation of how well changes accomplished during rehabilitation generalize to the real-life situation of the patient and family. The **Rehabilitation Outcome Questionnaire** collects data on client disability as experienced in the discharge environment. It also collects the crucial data for assessment of handicap.

The first issue which is addressed in the Rehabilitation Outcome Questionnaire is a survey of the individual's disability status in the discharge environment. Items are tied to goals that are typically important for brain-injured patients at different levels of care. For instance, key questions for coma patients relate to level of contact with the environment (Glasgow Coma Scale, Rancho Scale), any evidence of functional behaviour, expenditures for care, and preventable medical complications. For acute rehabilitation patients, physical and cognitive assistance in self-care and mobility ADLs as well as higher level community reintegration skills are measured. For community reintegration programmes, outcome assessment focuses on performance of those skills which the programme deemed as essential to support community readaptation. Ultimate status (institutionalization, employment etc.) is measured for all clients.

The Rehabilitation Outcome Questionnaire attempts to identify the most salient barriers to higher levels of performance. It contains items designed to identify reasons for failure to perform at the level observed upon completion of rehabilitation (e.g. skill not practical, equipment necessary to support performance not present, physical deterioration, neurobehavioural deficits).

The Rehabilitation Outcome Questionnaire provides objective data for the assessment of normative handicap by measuring the six survival roles in the WHO framework. The disability ratings of the questionnaire address the first three areas (orientation, physical independence, mobility). The questionnaire also contains items designed to assess the individual's engagement in work, school, leisure and recreational activities (occupation handicap) and his/her interpersonal and social relationships (social integration handicap). There is also a section on the financial impact of this disability for the patient and the family (economic handicap).

The most primary and most direct measure of handicap is also contained in the Rehabilitation Outcome Questionnaire. Handicap is primarily assessed by items relating to the degree of subjective burden or stress experienced by the patient and the family as a consequence of different forms of disability.

Phases

Follow-up is conducted in two phases. An extensive survey of disability and handicap is begun one month post-discharge. This survey is conducted by telephone. The procedure is repeated at 3 and 6 months. This phase of follow-up measures both proximal specific objectives (e.g. performance of a behaviour) and more ultimate or distal goals (e.g. employment/school, avoiding institutionalization).

The second phase of the follow-up focuses on current status in ultimate, distal goals. This will be conducted on yearly anniversaries of the discharge from rehabilitation. The aim here is to study long-term outcomes.

Automation

The information system is designed to be automated. Data are entered into local IBM PCs and designated terminals which transmit data electronically to the central data depository, an IBM 38. Current plans call for electronic transfer of data from the 38 to an IBM Personal System 2 Model 80 for analysis by SPSS or SAS.

12.4 UTILIZATION OF THE REIS

The primary purpose of the REIS is to gain knowledge regarding the effectiveness and efficiency of our rehabilitation programmes. We posit two principal methods for improving rehabilitation effectiveness: 1. distinguishing treatments that are effective in enhancing patient performance from those which are not; and 2. improving goal definition so that interventions are targeted towards reducing patient and family handicap in the discharge environment. The REIS is designed to answer a series of questions related to these issues. Each of these questions must be posed at both simple descriptive levels and at more complex levels of scientific inference.

Is the treatment effective in reducing disability?

At a simple but fundamental level, this question is, 'Do clients get better in the treatment setting?' Answers to questions of this nature are demanded by patients and families, referral sources, and payment sources (e.g. insurance companies and government agencies) and are needed for marketing. The CAIR answers this question by describing client disability at admission and discharge. Clients can be grouped according to admission disability level and major impairment types in the CAIR, permitting comparison of maximally comparable cases and reducing inappropriate judgements about effectiveness. Other important variables such as age, socioeconomic status, sex, nature and severity of initial injury, chronicity (interval between onset of injury and admission for rehabilitation), and client performance before the injury are readily available in the information system.

Yet the REIS is designed to go beyond this level. It is designed to answer questions relating to the efficacy of specific therapeutic interventions. By linking data on the hours of therapeutic services rendered towards goals in the Client Service Plan with actual client progress over time, it will be possible to inform programme personnel regarding the degree of change accomplished, expected time periods, and expected effort to achieve specific rehabilitation goals for various groups of rehabilitation clients. Case managers need this information even now, but the need for such information will become increasingly critical as we enter an era of managed health care in which rehabilitation facilities will be required by insurance companies to specify goals they will attain within prescribed cost of length or stay constraints.

Why?

Perhaps the most distinctive feature of the REIS is that it is designed to go beyond the question of whether disability reduction occurred to answer the question of why it occurred. Answering this question is critical, for without it there is no link to action or real answers to the question of what rehabilitative interventions are most effective. A client may, for instance, have failed to achieve a rehabilitative goal. To judge whether therapeutic effectiveness is even at issue one must know whether the stay was truncated because of an unforeseeable medical complication or unexpected end of funding. Moreover the efficacy of rehabilitative interventions depends upon the impairment basis of the person's disability. A second level of distinction is whether the change in patient performance is associated with therapeutic interventions. For instance, changes in patient performance due to changes in medication, clearing of an infection, or taking the person off bed rest must be distinguished from the effects of repeated therapeutic interventions. The effectiveness of therapeutic interventions involving compensatory activities or environmental modifications or techno-logical aids are likely to differ radically from the effectiveness of direct restorative strategies, depending on the impairments involved. In summary, the information system is designed to get as close as possible to the causes of client improvement or failure to improve.

Effectiveness of treatment cannot be fully established unless some comparison with a control group is possible. Control procedures using randomized assignment to treatment or non-treatment groups are likely to be neither ethical nor feasible. However, valid inferences regarding likely effectiveness and efficiency are sometimes possible using quasi-experimental research designs (Cook and Campbell, 1979). Here the diversity of the New Medico Head Injury System is an advan-tage. A variety of treatment strategies and philosophies can be found within New Medico, as within the field of head injury rehabilitation as a whole. We are optimistic about the likelihood of finding com-parison groups that will enable valid inference regarding the effec-tiveness and efficiency of various treatments.

Does the treatment effect generalize to the post discharge environment?

A major test of rehabilitative effectiveness is the extent to which skills acquired during training are actually employed in the discharge environment. Skills which are trained and reinforced by rehabilitative personnel are of little practical value if they are not employed in the discharge environment.

What are the reasons for failure of a skill obtained in rehabilitation to generalize? The Rehabilitation Outcome Questionnaire contains information on reasons for failure to generalize (e.g. change in discharge environment, medical complications, behaviour is not rein-forced, expected equipment not available). These data are a crucial component of programme evaluation for they can assist the clinical staff in designing methods to minimize these barriers to generalization. For example, programme staff may discover the need to structure the later portion of rehabilitation training to better approximate the conditions in the discharge environment. Staff may also decide that more effective family training is needed to increase the likelihood of generalization. Or it may be discovered that certain equipment or environmental modifications are the most cost-effective way of ensur-ing continued use of the trained skill.

What is the value of the disability reduction to the person?

This is the issue of handicap. The experience of two patients with comparable levels of objective performance may be quite different. One may express extreme distress while another may carry on without indication of undue distress. Such results are produced by differing levels of psychological adjustment as well as by different environmental demands (e.g. one person may have a large supportive family and adequate finances while the other loses what family he or she has and has no means of financial support).

Effective rehabilitation must anticipate these differences and address them *during* the training period. This can occur through targeted goal selection and through methods designed to reduce the subsequent experience of burden. By surveying the patient and family after discharge about the major sources of subjective burden, the Rehabilitation Outcome Questionnaire data can provide meaningful feedback to programme personnel to guide the process of improved goal selection and more targeted service delivery. For instance, it may be found that for a certain type of client, training for re-employment in the same job usually leads to subsequent failure and increased frustration, but training in leisure and prevocational skills leads more frequently to a stable living arrangement and enjoyable experiences. Or the contrary may be found. Regardless, the REIS has the data to answer such questions.

Prediction of outcomes

A major goal of the REIS is to predict rehabilitation outcomes. At one level this involves comparison of the clinical profile of a newly-admitted patient to outcomes of patients with similar profiles. Such data should assist in better goal definition, which will help to guide the outcome expectations of families.

Another type of prediction deals with assignment of a referred patient to a particular programme when more than one option exists. By matching the patient profile obtained from pre-admission data to outcomes achieved by the programmes which are considered options, selection of the programme with the highest probability of success for that specific case may be facilitated.

Both types of prediction can be done initially using simple averages for different client groups, but as data accumulate it will become possible to develop increasingly sophisticated predictive models using multivariate statistical methods. If we can develop valid and reliable predictive models, our understanding of factors driving effective rehabilitation will greatly advance.

Cost-effectiveness

The thrust of the REIS is improvement of cost-effectiveness via improvement of clinical effectiveness but, by linking information on client outcomes to financial factors, it permits direct study of the cost-effectiveness and efficiency of rehabilitative services. At a simple level, analysis of improvement per dollar or per day can yield insight into likely sources of programme efficiency or inefficiency. If groups can be identified that differ widely in cost but have few differences in impairments or disabilities, valid inference of cost-effectiveness becomes possible (Johnston, 1987). Here again this may be an issue unique to health care systems which are organized and funded like the US system.

Data on rehabilitation effectiveness and efficiency are invaluable to marketing and meet our obligation to use society's resources wisely. Rehabilitation professionals, insurance and governmental agencies, and consumers are in agreement that data on rehabilitation outcomes and cost-effectiveness are essential to determine the value of rehabilitation.

Administrative uses

The REIS is designed to meet a range of practical administrative needs to justify the cost of the system. The REIS contains information needed by programme case managers to communicate effectively with insurance and governmental agencies relative to patient status and goals, discharge planning, and eventual outcomes. REIS data will facilitate administrative activities such as projecting staffing needs, formulating budgets, and performing cost analyses. REIS data may help identify programme personnel who excel in certain types of patient management. The REIS provides all data required for programme evaluation and exceeds the programme evaluation standards of the Commission on Accreditation of Facilities (CARF, 1986a; b).

12.5 SUMMARY

In some fields of medicine, a hardware technology has been the chief vehicle of progress. Microbiology and the germ theory of disease rest on the microscope. Radiology is based on the X-ray machine and has progressed greatly with the CT scan and the MRI. But what is the instrument for progress in rehabilitation? It cannot be a single diagnostic device or hardware technology, for rehabilitation is too multifaceted. It is concerned with handicap and disability as much as with impairment and with social-environmental factors as well as characteristics of the client and family. Only a system that taps all these levels and domains can be an appropriate tool for overall progress in rehabilitation.

Progress in biomedical research today is rarely achieved by cheap, easy research. Great progress has been achieved in recent years, but only with sustained investigation by multidisciplinary teams over years of effort. The problems of rehabilitation after brain injury are so formidable that major progress is likely to be achieved only at a cost of major effort. It is our hope that the REIS will be an instrument for such progress. Success will hinge both on the completeness of implementation of the REIS and on how astutely we marshall its resources.

ACKNOWLEDGEMENTS

Preparation of this manuscript was funded by New Medico Associates, Inc. The authors thank the physicians and other rehabilitation professionals of the facilities of the New Medico Head Injury System for invaluable input during the design of the instruments described in this chapter.

REFERENCES

Ben-Yishay, Y., Rattok, J., Lakin, P. et al. (1985) Neuropsychologic Rehabilitation: Quest of a Holistic Approach. Semin. Neurol., 5, 252–59.

Ben-Yishay, Y., Silver, S., Piasetsky, E. and Rattok, J. (1987) Relationship Between Employability and Vocational Outcome After Intensive Holistic Cognitive Rehabilitation. J. Head Trauma Rehabil., 2(1), 35–48.

Bowers, S. and Marshall, L. (1980) Outcome of 200 Consecutive Cases of Severe Head Injury Treated in San Diego County: A Prospective Analysis. Neurosurg., 6(3), 237–42.

Braakman, R., Gelpke, G., Habbema, J., Maas, A. and Minderhoud, J. (1980) Systematic Selection of Prognostic Features in Patients with Severe Head Injury. Neurosurg., 6(4), 362–70.

Brooks, N. (1984) Closed Head Injury: Psychological, Social and Family Consequences, Oxford University Press, Oxford.

Brooks, N., Campsie, L., Symington, C. et al. (1986) The Five-Year Outcome of Severe Blunt Head Injury: A Relative's View. J. Neurol. Neurosurg. Psychiat., 49, 764–70.

Brooks, N., Campsie, L., Symington, C. et al. (1987) The Effects of Severe Head Injury on Patient and Relative within Seven Years of Injury. J. Head Trauma Rehabil., 2(3), 34–45.

Brown, M., Gordon, W. and Diller, L. (1982) Functional Assessment and Outcome Measurement: An Integrative Review in *Ann. Rev. Rehabil.* vol. 3 (E. Pan, T. Backer and C. Vash, eds), Springer, New York.

Commission on Accreditation of Rehabilitation Facilities (CARF) (1986a) *Program Evaluation in Inpatient Medical Rehabilitation Facilities*, Commission on Accreditation of Rehabilitation Facilities, Tucson.

Commission on Accreditation of Rehabilitation Facilities (CARF) (1986b) *Standards Manual for Facilities Serving People with Disabilities*, Commission on Accreditation of Rehabilitation Facilities, Tucson.

Cook, T. and Campbell, D. (1979) *Quasi-Experimentation: Design and Analysis Issues for Field Settings*, Rand McNally, Chicago.

Eames, P. and Wood, R. (1985) Rehabilitation After Severe Brain Injury: a Follow-up Study of a Behaviour Modification Approach. *J. Neurol. Neurosurg. Psychiat.*, **48**, 613–19.

Flanagan, J. (1982) Measurement of Quality of Life: Current State of the Art. *Arch. Phys. Med. Rehabil.*, **63**, 56–59.

Frey, W. (1984) Functional Assessment in the '80s: A Conceptual Enigma, A Technical Challenge in *Functional Assessment in Rehabilitation* (A. Halpern and M. Fuhrer, eds), Paul H. Brookes, Baltimore, pp. 9–43.

Fryer, L.J. and Haffey, W. (1987) Cognitive Rehabilitation and Community Readaptation: Outcomes from Two Program Models. *J. Head Trauma Rehabil.*, **2**(3) 67–79.

Gianotta, S., Weiner, J., and Karnaze, D. (1987) Prognosis and Outcome in Severe Head Injury in *Head Injury* 2nd edn (P.R. Cooper, ed.), Williams and Wilkins, Baltimore, pp. 464–87.

Gilchrist, E. and Wilkinson, M. (1979) Some Factors Determining the Prognosis in Young People with Severe Head Injuries. *Arch. Neurol.*, **36**, 355–59.

Granger, C. and Gresham, G. (1984) *Functional Assessment in Rehabilitation Medicine*, Williams and Wilkins, Baltimore.

Granger, C., Hamilton, B. and Sherwin, M. (1986) *Guide for the Use of the Uniform Data Set for Medical Rehabilitation*, Project Office: Department of Rehabilitation Medicine, Buffalo General Hospital, Buffalo.

Hagen, C., Malkmus, D. and Durham, P. (1974) *Levels of Cognitive Functioning.* Communications Disorders Service, Rancho Los Amigos Hospital, Los Angeles.

Halpern, A. and Fuhrer, M. (1984) *Functional Assessment in Rehabilitation*, Paul H. Brookes, Baltimore.

Hart, T. and Hayden, M. (1986) Issues in the Evaluation of Rehabilitation Effects in *Neurotrauma: Treatment, Rehabilitation and Related Issues* (M. Miner and K. Wagner, eds), Butterworth, Boston, pp. 197–212.

Jennett, B. and Bond, M. (1975) Assessment of Outcome After Severe Brain Damage, *Lancet*, **i**, 480–84.

Jennett, B., Snoek, J., Bond, M. and Brooks, N. (1981) Disability After Severe Head Injury: Observations on the Use of the Glasgow Outcome Scale. *J. Neurol. Neurosurg. Psychiat.*, **44**, 285–93.

Jennett, B., Teasdale, G., Braakman, R. *et al.* (1979) Prognosis of Patients with Severe Head Injury. *Neurosurgery*, **4**(4), 283–89.

Jennett, B., Teasdale, G., Braakman, R. *et al.* (1976) Predicting Outcome in Individual Patients After Severe Head Injury, *Lancet*, **i**, 1031–35.

Johnston, M.V. (1983) *The Costs and Effectiveness of Stroke Rehabilitation: Measurement and Prediction*, PhD dissertation, Claremont Graduate School, Claremont, CA.

Johnston, M.V. (1987) Cost-Benefit Methodologies in Rehabilitation in *Rehabilitation*

Outcomes: Analysis and Measurement (M.J. Fuhrer, ed.), Paul H. Brookes, Baltimore, pp 99–114.

Kottke, F. (1982) Philosophic Considerations of Quality of Life for the Disabled. *Arch. Phys. Med. Rehabil.*, **63**, 60–62.

Levin, H. (1985) Part II, Neurobehavioural Recovery in *Central Nervous System Trauma Status Report* (M. Becker and J. Povlishock, eds), National Institutes of Health, Washington, pp. 281–299.

Levin, H., Benton, A. and Grossman, R. (1982) *Neurobehavioural Consequences of Closed Head Injury*, Oxford Univeristy Press, New York.

Lezak, M.D. (1987) *Neurological Assessment*, 2nd edn, Oxford University Press, New York.

Livingston, M. (1987) Head Injury: the Relative's Response. *Brain Injury*, 1(1), 33–39.

Livingston, M., Brooks, D. and Bond, M. (1985) Patient Outcome in the Year Following Severe Head Injury and Relative's Social Psychiatric and Social Functioning. *J. Neurol. Neurosurg. Psychiat.*, **48**, 876–81.

McKinlay, W., Brooks, D., Bond, M. *et al.* (1981) The Short-Term Outcome of Severe Blunt Head Injury as Reported by Relatives of the Injured Persons. *J. Neurol. Neurosurg. Psychiat.*, **44**, 527–33.

Nagi, S. (1969) *Disability and Rehabilitation: Legal, Clinical and Self Concepts and Measurement*, Ohio State University Press, Columbus.

Najenson, T., Groswasser, Z., Stern, M. *et al.* (1975) Prognostic Factors in Rehabilitation After Severe Head Injury. *Scand. J. Rehabil. Med.*, **7**, 101–05.

Najenson, T., Sazbon, L., Fizelzon, J. *et al.* (1978) Recovery of Communicative Functions After Prolonged Traumatic Coma. *Scand. J. Rehabil. Med.*, **10**, 15–21.

Oddy, M., Coughlin, T., Tyerman, A. and Jenkins, D. (1985) Social Adjustment After Closed Head Injury: A Further Follow-Up Seven Years After Injury. *J. Neurol., Neurosurg. Psychiat.*, **48**, 564–68.

Prigitano, G., Fordyce, D., Zeiner, H. *et al.* (1984) Neuropsychological Rehabilitation After Closed Head Injury in Young Adults. *J. Neurol. Neurosurg. Psychiat.*, **47**, 505–13.

Scherzer, B. (1986) Rehabilitation Following Severe Head Trauma: Results of a Three-Year Program. *Arch. Phys. Med. Rehabil.*, **67**, 366–73.

Thomsen, I. (1984) Late Outcome of Very Severe Blunt Head Trauma: 10–15 Year Second Follow-Up. *J. Neurol. Neurosurg. Psychiat.*, **47**, 260–68.

Treischmann, R. (1974) Coping With a Disability: A Sliding Scale of Goals. *Arch. Phys. Med. Rehabil.*, **55**, 556–60.

Weddell, R., Oddy, M. and Jenkins, D. (1980) Social Adjustment after Rehabilitation: A Two Year Follow-up of Patients with Severe Head Injury. *Psychol. Med.*, **10**, 257–63.

WHO (1980) International Classification of Impairments, Disabilities and Handicaps. Geneva, World Health Organization.

Wood, P.H.N. (1975) Classification of Impairment and Handicap Document WHO–ICDO–REVCOMF–75.15. Geneva, WHO.

Wood, R.Ll (1987) Neuropsychological Assessment in Brain Injury Rehabilitation in *Advances in Rehabilitation* (M.G. Eisenburg and R.C. Grzesiak, eds), Springer, New York.

Index